Acad... l

D0492299

The Insider's Guide
to the MRCS Clinical
Examination

The Insider's Guide to the MRCS Clinical Examination

JONATHAN M FISHMAN
BA (Hons), MA (Cantab), BM BCh (Oxon), MRCS (Eng), DOHNS (RCS Eng)
ENT Specialist Registrar, The John Radcliffe Hospital, Oxford

VIVIAN A ELWELL
BA (Hons), MA (Cantab), MB BS, MRCS
Neurosurgery Specialist Registrar, Charing Cross Hospital, London

RAJAT CHOWDHURY
BSc (Hons), MSc (Lond), MA (Oxon), BM BCh (Oxon), MRCS
Radiology Specialist Registrar, Southampton General Hospital, Southampton

And all Managing Directors of Insider Medical Ltd

Foreword by
NIGEL D MENDOZA
*Consultant Neurosurgeon, Imperial College Healthcare NHS Trust
Honorary Clinical Lecturer, Imperial College School of Medicine,
London*

Radcliffe Publishing
Oxford • New York

Radcliffe Publishing Ltd
18 Marcham Road
Abingdon
Oxon OX14 1AA
United Kingdom

www.radcliffe-oxford.com
Electronic catalogue and worldwide online ordering facility.

British Library Cataloguing in Publication Data

A catalogue record for this book is available from the British Library.

ISBN-13: 978 1 84619 297 5

Typeset by Pindar NZ, Auckland, New Zealand
Printed and bound by TJI Digital, Padstow, Cornwall, UK

Contents

Foreword

The MRCS Clinical Examination is the final requirement for obtaining the professional qualification for the Intercollegiate Membership of the Royal College of Surgeons. This Membership allows the transition from doctor to surgeon and a career in higher surgical training. The standardised clinical examination requires candidates to demonstrate their ability when examining patients, with effective and clear communication.

The authors should be commended on producing a book that covers all clinical sections of the examination in such a concise, comprehensive and structured manner. The approach adopted is to focus the candidate's revision in a productive way and address the various conditions that they will encounter. This study guide will serve as the candidate's personal tutor, working closely with them, prompting and providing pointers to improve their examination technique. It includes dozens of clinical scenarios, demonstrating how to examine specific systems and avoid common mistakes. In addition, the candidate can improve their communication skills, which are an integral part of this examination.

This book complements the Insider Medical MRCS Clinical Course. It simulates the actual test conditions by providing sample cases and answers, coupling identification of weaknesses and strengths. This book will also prove to be extremely valuable for the new-style MRCS OSCE.

The wide-ranging nature of surgery can be overwhelming, and sometimes it may be difficult to 'separate the wood from the trees.' However, as Robert Frost wrote:

Two roads diverged in a wood, and I –
I took the one less travelled by,
And that has made all the difference.

This book enables successful revision with clear targets to pass the MRCS Clinical Examination.

I wish you all the best in your endeavours. Good luck!

Nigel D Mendoza
Consultant Neurosurgeon, Imperial College Healthcare NHS Trust
Honorary Clinical Lecturer, Imperial College School of Medicine,
London
August 2008

About the authors

Jonathan M Fishman BA (Hons), MA (Cantab), BM BCh (Oxon), MRCS (Eng), DOHNS (RCS Eng)

Jonathan is an Oxford Specialist Registrar in ENT and a member of the Royal College of Surgeons. He graduated with a First Class Honours Degree in Natural Sciences from Sidney Sussex College, University of Cambridge, and completed his clinical training at St John's College, University of Oxford. He has held posts in Accident and Emergency, ENT, general surgery and neurosurgery, as part of the surgical rotation at St Mary's Hospital, Imperial College, London.

Jonathan has extensive teaching experience and is the primary author of three undergraduate medical textbooks, including the highly successful *History Taking in Medicine and Surgery* (Pastest Publishing, 2005). He spent part of his medical training at both Harvard University and the NASA Space Center.

Jonathan was awarded Taylor and Howard-Agg Scholarships at Sidney Sussex College, Cambridge, and has been awarded the highly prestigious title of 'Lifelong Honorary Scholar' by the University of Cambridge, for academic excellence. He has been awarded a fellowship from the British Association of Plastic Surgeons for research at NASA, and from Cambridge University for research at Harvard University. He is committed to a career in academic ENT, with a strong emphasis on teaching and career development.

Vivian A Elwell BA (Hons), MA (Cantab), MB BS, MRCS

Currently working as a Specialist Registrar in Neurosurgery, Vivian has held posts in Accident and Emergency, orthopaedics, neurosurgery and general surgery with the surgical rotation at St Mary's Hospital, Imperial College, London.

She is an author of a best-selling undergraduate textbook, *Essential OSCE Topics for Medical and Surgical Finals* (Radcliffe Publishing, 2008). She taught clinical skills to medical students and doctors, and was an anatomy demonstrator at the Imperial College School of Medicine, London. She also served on the Imperial College School of Medicine Curriculum Development Committee.

Vivian's awards include the Swinford Edward Silver Medal Prize for her OSCE Examination, the Columbia University Research Fellowship at Columbia College of Physicians and Surgeons in New York City, the Columbia University King's Crown Gold and Silver Medal Awards, the Kathrine Dulin Folger Cancer Research Fellowship and the 'Who's Who of Young Scientists Prize.'

She earned a Bachelor's degree in biological sciences at Columbia College, Columbia University, and an MA from the University of Cambridge. She gained Bachelor of Medicine and Bachelor of Surgery degrees from the Imperial College School of Medicine, and is a member of the Royal College of Surgeons.

Rajat Chowdhury BSc (Hons), MSc (Lond), MA (Oxon), BM BCh (Oxon), MRCS

Rajat is a Specialist Registrar in Radiology and is a member of the Royal College of Surgeons. He was awarded an Honours degree in biological science from University College London, and completed his medical studies at Oxford University, the Mayo Clinic and Harvard University. He then trained on the surgical rotation at St Mary's Hospital, Imperial College, London, and held posts in Accident and Emergency, orthopaedics and trauma, cardiothoracic surgery, general surgery, and plastic surgery.

Rajat has a diverse teaching record. He has taught clinical medicine to students and doctors in Oxford and London, and has tutored biochemistry and genetics to undergraduate students at Oxford University. He was an anatomy demonstrator at the Imperial College School of Medicine, London, and was President of the Queen's College Medical Society, Oxford, and of the Hugh Cairns Surgical Society.

Rajat's academic awards include Oxford University's Bristol Myers Squibb Prize in Cardiology, the Radcliffe Infirmary Prize for Surgery, the GlaxoSmithKline Medical Fellowship, the Warren Scholarship for

Paediatric Studies at the University of Toronto, and the Exhibition Award to Harvard University. He is committed to a career in interventional and academic radiology. He has successfully completed Part 1 of the FRCR examinations, and is the lead author of the forthcoming undergraduate textbook, *Radiology at a Glance* (Blackwell-Wiley Publishing).

Preface

This book is devoted to the MRCS Clinical Examination, successful completion of which must be attained before full membership of one of the Royal Colleges of Surgeons of Great Britain and Ireland can be conferred upon an individual.

The standard requirements for passing the clinical examination should not be underestimated. Success, as with any other clinical examination, requires a solid working knowledge and a well-rehearsed examination technique. A precise, structured and systematic routine is paramount. This technique ensures that key steps of the clinical examination are not accidentally omitted, and under the pressure of the examination it provides a defined starting point and framework for any case that one may encounter.

It is a commonly held view that when candidates fail this examination, this is due to a lack of knowledge. However, in our experience, most candidates do possess sufficient knowledge to pass the examination, but lack a systematic and structured approach, which results in hesitancy. It is all too easy to become overly conscious of the presence of the examiners and to jump from one aspect of the clinical examination to another, without clear structure and organisation. This creates a bad impression, and the candidate loses sight of the main problem. The psychological impact of a bad station can be devastating for the doctor and, given the nature of the MRCS clinical examination, it can significantly affect their performance on subsequent stations. However, a coherent and well-rehearsed examination routine will not only ensure exam success, but will also mean that the candidate knows how to proceed when faced with difficult cases which they may not have encountered previously.

In the MRCS examination, perhaps more than in any other examination, time pressure and emotions can often hinder performance. This book will discuss and explain the commonly encountered clinical examinations, and these will be instrumental in guiding doctors in their revision. A systematic, logical and prescriptive approach will be adopted. The book will also focus on communication skills and enable doctors to communicate effectively both with patients and with fellow colleagues.

This book is based on our highly successful 'Insider Medical MRCS Examination Clinical Course', and aims to equip the candidate with a systematic approach, as well as our 'top tips' for the cases commonly encountered in the MRCS Clinical Examination. As well as providing examination routines approved by many College examiners, we shall also offer 'Insider' tips on how to pass the examination. We have a wealth and breadth of experience of teaching at both undergraduate and postgraduate levels, and have identified mistakes that are commonly made by many candidates. Our aim is to facilitate the pathway for a novice clinician to pass this challenging examination with ease.

We are confident that this book can lead future surgeons on the road to success. It is our intention to assist doctors in passing the MRCS Clinical Examination, and to turn the common perception of this from being a 'mission impossible' to being an achievable result. Finally, through this book we hope to attain our ultimate goal of preparing future surgeons for the challenges of mastering their art.

Jonathan M Fishman
Vivian A Elwell
Rajat Chowdhury
August 2008

List of abbreviations

#	Fracture
AAA	Abdominal aortic aneurysm
ABPI	Ankle to brachial pressure index
ACJ	Acromioclavicular joint
ACL	Anterior cruciate ligament
AF	Atrial fibrillation
AP	Antero-posterior
AS	Ankylosing spondylitis
ASIS	Anterior superior iliac spine
BCC	Basal-cell carcinoma
BP	Blood pressure
BR	Brachioradialis
CABG	Coronary artery bypass graft
CMV	Cytomegalovirus
COPD	Chronic obstructive pulmonary disease
CSF	Cerebrospinal fluid
CT	Computed tomography
CXR	Chest X-ray
DIPJ	Distal interphalangeal joint
DVT	Deep vein thrombosis
EBV	Epstein–Barr virus
ECRL	Extensor carpi radialis longus
ENT	Ear, nose and throat
EPL	Extensor pollicis longus
ESR	Erythrocyte sedimentation rate
FCU	Flexor carpi ulnaris
FDP	Flexor digitorum profundus

FDS	Flexor digitorum superficialis
FFD	Fixed flexion deformity
FPL	Flexor pollicis longus
HIV	Human immunodeficiency virus
IPJ	Interphalangeal joint
LMN	Lower motor neuron
MCPJ	Metacarpophalangeal joint
MRC	Medical Research Council
MRCS	Membership of the Royal College of Surgeons
MRI	Magnetic resonance imaging
MTP	Metatarsophalangeal joint
n	Nerve
OA	Osteoarthritis
PCA	Patient-controlled analgesia
PE	Pulmonary embolism
PIPJ	Proximal interphalangeal joint
RA	Rheumatoid arthritis
RIF	Right iliac fossa
SCC	Squamous-cell carcinoma
SFJ	Sapheno-femoral junction
SIJ	Sacroiliac joint
SLE	Systemic lupus erythematosus
SVC	Superior vena cava
TB	Tuberculosis
TED	thromboembolic deterrent stockings
TRAM	Transverse rectus abdominis myocutaneous
UMN	Upper motor neuron
USS	Ultrasound scan

To all our families, colleagues and patients without whom
Insider Medical Ltd would not be possible.

Introducing the MRCS clinical exam: the Insider's guide to success

May I introduce Mr/Miss . . .

The final test

Successful completion of the written and viva voce components of the Intercollegiate MRCS examination allows passage to the MRCS Clinical Examination, which is the final gateway for admission to one of the surgeons' clubs. This transition is a major landmark in your career, as it recognises your demonstrated commitment to surgery. The clinical examination differs markedly from the other parts of the MRCS in that it is the surgical art more than the science that is being tested. This examination is designed to assess your ability to apply your trade to your patients with skill and integrity.

The clinical exam consists of four clinical bays lasting 15 minutes each, and divided into:

1 superficial lesions
2 the musculoskeletal and neurological systems
3 the circulatory system
4 the abdomen and trunk.

A surgeon's communication skills are also formally tested in two 15-minute bays:

1 information gathering
2 information giving.

Each bay is usually examined by two surgeons, typically in a specialty different from their own. The underlying qualities that are therefore being examined are the professionalism in your approach to history taking, physical examination, differential diagnosis formulation and management planning.

The marking scheme

The specific areas where points are awarded can be categorised as follows:

Attitudes
- Introduction.
- Patient interaction.
- Patient courtesy.
- Professional interaction.

Clinical skills
- Gentleness of handling.
- Organisation of approach.
- General assessment.
- System-specific inspection.
- System-specific palpation.
- Other relevant assessments.
- Identification of clinical signs.

Knowledge
- Differential diagnosis.
- Management plan.

Getting it right

It is clear from the marking scheme that most points are awarded for your general behaviour, conduct and systematic approach. Many candidates make the mistake of spending all their preparation time focusing on the 'Knowledge' section, and are often careless and lack confidence in their approach. This is frequently the cause of an unsuccessful outcome. You should view taking the clinical exam in the same way as taking the driving test. In the driving test candidates make a definite display of the 'mirror, signal, manoeuvre' routine for the examiner, and similarly it is vital to pay attention to basic protocols such as hand washing before and after seeing each patient, ensuring that appropriate patient introductions take place, obtaining verbal consent, etc.

Practice makes perfect

As with all exams, meticulous preparation is the key. Many candidates spend most of their time visiting various clinics, hungry for common and esoteric pathology. However, it is undoubtedly better to work with a fellow candidate and draw up a list of all the common cases for each bay. Then, as a team, you can diligently focus on practising and critiquing each other's systematic physical examinations until you have perfected the ultimate in slick technique. It is only through practice that attention to handwashing and clarity of patient instructions becomes automatic. The mechanics of the physical examination should become reflex in nature, and you can then optimise your efforts in eliciting the signs to confidently generate appropriate differential diagnoses with ease. Physical examinations for the purposes of the MRCS clinical exam should take no longer than 90 seconds, and you must be prepared for interruptions by the examiners and then continue unperturbed by these. Under examination pressure, these reflex responses will be lifelines for displaying your core competencies with confidence, and will thereby carry you safely through to success in what may seem like a baffling case.

The mind game

The most important concept that you should consider is your mindset. It is important to realise that examiners are looking to see whether you possess the so-called 'Registrar quality.' Therefore you should approach the exam wearing your 'Registrar hat', and demonstrate appropriate levels of confidence, gravitas, maturity, safe decision-making and management skills, in addition to your core surgical knowledge. Successful candidates are those who possess flair and finesse, deliver safe logical work-ups, and in essence portray themselves as a contender for the role of a consultant's deputy.

The look

The impact of a candidate's appearance and presentation must not be underestimated. Some basic but golden nuggets for portraying yourself as a responsible, respectable, knowledgeable and safe surgeon are as follows:

▶ Female candidates: neutral suit and blouse, minimal jewellery and make-up, long hair tied back, comfortable shoes, antiperspirant, and perhaps subtle perfume. *Remember that you're the surgical reg!*

3

▶ Male candidates: grey or dark suit, white or blue shirt, no crested or club/college ties, recent smart haircut, no jewellery (except wedding band), clean shoes, antiperspirant, and perhaps subtle aftershave. *Remember that you're the surgical reg!*

The dress rehearsal

Revision courses that simulate the exam are excellent for giving you a dry run. They are best done when you are nearing the end of your preparation, to highlight areas of refinement to raise your game. You can learn both from your own mock exam experience and from viewing others in action. This is a time to allow others to critique your performance and point out any bad habits to which you may be oblivious. To get the most from the mock exam experience, you should attend in the attire you ultimately intend to wear, both to ensure that it is comfortable and also to identify the best pockets for your tools, such as your stethoscope.

The night before

Preparation begins long before the big day. Make sure that you are in possession of the following pieces of equipment:
▶ stethoscope
▶ short (15 cm) ruler
▶ tape measure
▶ pen torch
▶ tongue depressor
▶ opaque tube (e.g. Smartie tube) for transillumination
▶ tourniquet (for varicose veins)
▶ hat pins (for neurological examination)
▶ a piece of card for the ulnar nerve examination
▶ goniometer.

It is always better to take your own equipment to the exam if possible, as this is what you will be most familiar with. However, try not to overload your pockets to the extent that they look unsightly, or you are unable to find something if you need it. Tendon hammers and any other pieces of equipment that you may require will be provided during the exam. Make sure that you know how to use a goniometer, for instance, if you are handed one in the exam.

You should arrange your travel itinerary as soon as you receive notification of your exam centre and date, and male candidates should get a smart haircut the week preceding the exam. On the evening before the big day, you should recheck your itinerary and then prepare your clothes, shoes and bag (including an antiperspirant if you are prone to anxiety-related sweating). You should probably not try out a new restaurant or hit the town, but instead set your alarm clock slightly earlier than you think you comfortably need, and then get a good night's rest.

The big day

When you awake on the morning of the exam, check the travel updates first, get washed and dressed and make sure that you have breakfast. Before you leave, look in the mirror and ask yourself 'Do I look like a surgical registrar?' The answer should most definitely be yes.

You must remember that you are potentially on display to the examiners before you arrive at the exam centre. They may be travelling on the same mode of public transport and may be looking out for exam candidates. You should therefore conduct yourself professionally and be polite and courteous at all times. So remember to leave home as the surgical reg!

In the exam itself . . .

- You cannot be too polite and courteous to patients.
- You must use the handwash gel before and after every patient.
- Make sure that you listen to the examiner's instructions very carefully, and only examine what you have been asked to examine. For example, if you are asked to 'examine the patient's thyroid status', then after general inspection, start with the hands. On the other hand, if you are asked to 'examine the thyroid gland', go straight to the neck. If you are at all unclear about what is required of you, do not be afraid to ask the examiner to repeat or rephrase the question.
- Try to maintain eye contact with the examiners, keep things simple, and always speak slowly, clearly and decisively.
- Most examiners prefer it if you talk out loud as you go along and then summarise your findings (both positive and negative) at the end. The advantages of talking to the examiners as you go along are twofold. First, it enables the examiners to understand your train of thought. Secondly, if you save everything up for the end, you risk forgetting something, and if the bell goes beforehand, then you have missed your golden opportunity to shine!

▶ The examiners will often direct you, and you should follow their instructions or take their hint if they are moving you towards a different discussion.

▶ If you have a difficult case that you don't feel went well, you must put your ruminations on hold and continue unperturbed. Remember that a surgical registrar remains unflustered and provides inspiration and leadership to others in situations of crisis.

The key to success

If you enter the exam looking, feeling and thinking like a surgical registrar, you're moments away from introducing yourself as 'Mr . . .' or 'Miss . . .' and joining that coveted club!

All the very best of luck!

SECTION A

The introduction

When you approach any patient in the exam, do not forget to first wash your hands with the hand gel. Then, as a general principle, remember the three P's:

▶ permission
▶ position
▶ pain.

It is worth memorising an introductory sentence before approaching any patient in the exam. A useful sentence for introducing yourself and gaining consent might be:

> *'Good morning/afternoon. Thank you for coming along today. I'm one of the surgical doctors taking part in the examination today. May I examine you please?'*

Consent has then been obtained. To examine a patient without having first obtained consent would constitute battery, resulting in an automatic fail.

Always gain adequate exposure of the area that you wish to examine, and position the patient appropriately.

Always ask the patient whether they have any pain before you lay a hand on them.

You may then begin to inspect around the patient for clues (walking aids, truss, etc.).

There are two ways to summarise your findings at the end of the examination. The first method is to be bold, state the diagnosis and then list the features in favour of the diagnosis. For example:

> *'This patient has a toxic multinodular goitre, as evidenced by . . .'*

This method is fine if your diagnosis is correct, but if you are wrong it can have deleterious effects.

The alternative and often preferred method is to summarise your relevant clinical findings (positive and negative) and then conclude with a sentence such as:

> *'This is consistent with a diagnosis of . . .' or*

> *'These findings support a diagnosis of . . .'*

Superficial lesions: head, neck, breast and cutaneous lesions

Approach to any lump (or cutaneous lesion)

1 **Introduce yourself** to the patient and wash your hands.

2 **Look.**

The rule of S's:

▶ Site (distance in cm from nearest joint, anatomical triangle of neck, etc.).

▶ Size (diameter in cm).

▶ Shape (hemispherical, lobulated, etc.).

▶ Surface and smoothness – overlying punctum, smooth/bosselated surface.

▶ Skin overlying – skin changes/colour, scars (with an overlying scar think of an implantation dermoid, pyogenic granuloma or recurrence following surgery).

▶ Surroundings – other lumps, satellite nodules.

▶ Special characteristics – e.g. moves with swallowing, protrusion of tongue.

▶ Edge – well-defined/ill-defined edge/border.

3 **Palpate.**

Tenderness – ask 'Is it tender if I press it?'

Temperature – use the back of the hand (which is more sensitive).

Try to ascertain which layer the lump is in. (Can you pinch the skin overlying the lump, or can you move the skin over it? Does the lump move with the skin?)

For skin lesions, is it flush with the skin, or is it raised?

Tense/contract the underlying muscle:

▶ Test for mobility/fixity of the lump at rest in two orthogonal planes.

▶ Then ask the patient to contract the underlying muscle.

▶ Ask yourself whether the lump is more or less prominent.

▶ Ask yourself whether the lump is more or less mobile with the muscle contracted (in two planes).

Consistency – soft, firm, hard or bony hard.

Fluctuance – in two planes at right angles to each other (Paget's sign).

Regional lymph node status (NEVER forget this!)

Insider's tip

As a general rule, if the lump:

- retains mobility and is more prominent when the underlying muscle is contracted, the *lump is superficial to muscle*
- is more prominent but less mobile when the underlying muscle is contracted, the *lump is attached to fascia or superficial surface of muscle*
- is less mobile and less prominent when the underlying muscle is contracted, the *lump is within muscle*
- is less mobile and less prominent when the underlying muscle is contracted, the *lump is deep to muscle.*

The one exception to the rule occurs when there is a *defect* in the muscle. In such cases, although the lump arises in, or deep to, the muscle, it appears more prominent when the muscle is contracted (e.g. ruptured muscle fibres as in a torn long head of biceps, incisional hernias, divarication of the rectus sheath, etc.).

Extra tests – cough impulse, reducibility, compressibility, thrill, transillumination, pulsatility and expansility.

4 **Percuss.**

5 **Auscultate** – bruits, bowel sounds.

6 **Surrounding neurovascular status** – distal pulses, sensation.

7 **Ask the patient some questions/take a full history.**

8 **Assess the impact of the condition on the patient's life.**

9 **Assess the patient's fitness for surgery.**

10 **Thank the patient and wash your hands.**

11 **Summarise and offer your differential diagnosis.**

Note: If you suspect lymphadenopathy, do not forget to check the drainage sites and check other areas for lymphadenopathy (cervical, axilla, epitrochlear, inguinal region, spleen, liver).

For example, in a patient with inguinal lymphadenopathy, the areas that drain to the inguinal lymph nodes include the lower limbs, the lower anterior abdominal wall (below the level of the umbilicus), and the perineum, anus, buttocks, scrotum and external genitalia, but not the testes, which drain to the para-aortic lymph nodes. All of these areas need to be checked carefully for sites of infections, or primary carcinomas.

Likewise, in a patient with a pre-auricular lymph node mimicking a parotid swelling, do not forget to check the scalp carefully for a squamous-cell carcinoma or malignant melanoma hidden within the hair!

Examination of the parotid lump

1 **Introduce yourself** to the patient and **wash your hands.**

2 **Look** at both sides and proceed as above. Look carefully for scars.

3 **Palpate** – proceed as above. Ask whether the lump is tender before feeling it, and ask the patient to tense the underlying masseter muscle by requesting them to clench their jaw. Test for fixity. Define the characteristics of the lump, as you would for any other lump.

4 **Examine the regional lymph nodes.**
Look for evidence of scalp infection, or a primary carcinoma hidden in the scalp (if you suspect a pre-auricular lymph node).

5 **Check the oral cavity/oropharynx** – use two tongue depressors and ask the patient to move their tongue to the right, to the left, place it on the roof of the mouth and then say Aaaaah, so that you can look at the palate and fauces.
 ▶ Examine the site of the parotid duct opposite the upper second molar teeth (pus, calculus).
 ▶ Examine the fauces for evidence of medialisation of the tonsils from a mass in the deep lobe of the parotid.
 ▶ Try to express pus out the parotid duct by gently massaging the gland and looking at the duct orifice.
 ▶ Offer to bimanually palpate the parotid gland (feel the duct and gland), although the clinical value of this is limited compared with the submandibular gland, because the parotid lies behind the anterior edge of the masseter muscle and the vertical ramus of the mandible.

6 **Check the integrity of the VII (facial) nerve** – ask the patient to 'Raise your eyebrows', 'Shut your eyes tight', 'Blow out your cheeks', 'Whistle', 'Show me your teeth', 'Grimace', and check taste sensation in the anterior two-thirds of the tongue.

7 **Check the contralateral side.**

8 **Offer a full ENT examination.**

9 **Differential diagnosis.**
   Bear in mind that not every lump in the parotid region is a parotid gland swelling, and it may be related to:
   - skin (sebaceous cyst, fungating squamous-cell carcinoma)
   - subcutaneous tissue (lipoma, dermoid cyst)
   - muscle (masseter muscle hypertrophy)
   - facial nerve (neuroma)
   - lymphatics (pre-auricular lymph node)
   - bone (winging of mandible, transverse process atlas/axis)
   - salivary tissue, i.e. the parotid gland itself (which may be benign or malignant).

10 **Thank the patient and wash your hands.**

11 **Summarise and offer your differential diagnosis.**
   In summary, for a lesion in the parotid region, do not forget to:
   - check the regional lymph node status
   - check the integrity of the facial nerve
   - look in the mouth.

Examination of the submandibular region

1 Introduce yourself to the patient and wash your hands.

2 Look at both sides and proceed as above. Inspect carefully for scars and evidence of marginal mandibular nerve weakness.

3 Palpate the gland – proceed as above, tense the floor of the mouth (by requesting the patient to push their tongue against the roof of their mouth), and ask the patient to contract the sternocleidomastoid muscle to determine the relationship of the swelling to the muscle.

4 Look inside the mouth at the submandibular duct orifice (pus, calculus).
   Check the lymphatic drainage sites and look for evidence of dental infection, or a primary carcinoma in the mouth (submental and submandibular lymph nodes drain the oral cavity).

5 Offer a bimanual palpation (ask for gloves!). Submandibular glands are ballottable, whereas submandibular lymph nodes are not.
   Try to express pus out of the submandibular duct by massaging the gland and looking at the duct orifice.

6 Test tongue sensation (lingual nerve) and mobility (hypoglossal nerve) – malignant infiltration of nerves.

7 Examine the regional lymph nodes.

8 Check the contralateral side and the parotid glands.

9 Offer a full ENT examination.

10 Differential diagnosis.
   ▶ Skin (sebaceous cyst, fungating squamous-cell carcinoma).
   ▶ Subcutaneous tissue (lipoma, dermoid cyst).
   ▶ Lymphatics (submandibular lymph node).
   ▶ Nerve (neuroma).
   ▶ Salivary tissue, i.e. submandibular gland enlargement

(benign conditions such as calculus/sialolithiasis, sialadenitis, sialectasis and sialosis, benign neoplasms such as pleomorphic adenoma, malignant neoplasms such as mucoepidermoid tumours).

11 **Thank the patient and wash your hands.**

12 **Summarise and offer your differential diagnosis.**

Examination of the neck and thyroid gland

1 **Introduce yourself to the patient and wash your hands.**
Position the chair well away from the wall so that you can easily get behind it.

Ask the patient to unfasten their top buttons to expose the upper chest so that a midline sternotomy scar is not missed (retrosternal goitre surgery), and also so that distended/engorged veins can be seen (SVC obstruction).

Ask whether there is any tenderness before palpating.

2 **Look** around the bed for clues, and look at the patient as a whole (thyroid status).

3 **Ask for a glass of water** if there is not one visible.

4 **Assess hoarseness of the voice** by asking the patient to count from 1 to 10.

Ask them to take in a deep breath, and listen for stridor.

5 **Inspect the neck from the front, sides and back.**
  ▶ Are there any obvious neck swellings or visible scars? Comment whether the lump is in the anterior or posterior triangle.
  ▶ Ask the patient to open their mouth and stick out their tongue. If the swelling is a thyroglossal duct cyst, the upward tug when the patient protrudes their tongue is unmistakable. Note that the mouth must be open at the commencement of the test when the swelling is grasped. You may check for a lingual thyroid simultaneously at the base of the tongue while the patient's mouth is open.
  ▶ Ask the patient to take a sip of water, hold it in their mouth and swallow when you instruct them to, with their chin slightly elevated. Does the lump move with swallowing? If it does, this implies that the swelling is thyroid related.

6 **Palpate from behind.**
Explain to the patient what you are about to do, and then move behind them.

Ask again whether it is tender.

19

Palpate from behind, but when you start to press on the thyroid look at the patient's face for signs of discomfort. Slightly flex the patient's head. Put one hand flat on one lobe and push it towards the midline. This will make the other side more prominent.

Check the following:

▶ Tenderness.
▶ Temperature.
▶ Ask the patient to swallow again (this time ask yourself whether you can get below the thyroid gland when the patient swallows. If you can, this excludes retrosternal extension).
▶ Size of goitre.
▶ Consistency (soft, firm or hard; uniform or varied).
▶ Single, diffuse or multiple swellings.
▶ Surface – smooth or nodular (any there any prominent nodules?)
▶ Also check mobility and relation to surroundings (skin, trachea, muscle and carotid artery) for fixity, displacement and infiltration:
   — Gently pinch the skin over the thyroid to check for fixity.
   — Check for fixation to the trachea (in two planes) and for tracheal displacement/deviation.
   — Check the relationship of the gland to the sternocleidomastoid muscle (ask the patient to look to one side and then gently push their chin down on the volar aspect of your wrist).
   — Assess the carotid artery pulsations (Berry's sign).

Do not forget to examine the regional lymph node groups in a systematic manner from behind (submental, submandibular, deep cervical chain including the jugulodigastric group, supraclavicular, superficial cervical chain, pre- and post-auricular, occipital, pre-tracheal and pre-laryngeal groups).

7 **Percuss** from the sternum upwards to test for retrosternal extension.

8 **Auscultate** for a thyroid bruit (while the patient holds their breath).

9 **Finishing statement:**

'To complete my examination, I would like to assess the patient's thyroid status and ask them some questions. In addition, I would like to check this patient's vocal cords by flexible laryngoscopy.'

You can also offer to perform Pemberton's test/sign. Ask the patient to elevate their arms above their head for 1 minute, and look for congestion, cyanosis, stridor and distended neck veins, as a sign of a large retrosternal goitre.

10 **Thank the patient and wash your hands.**

11 **Summarise and offer your differential diagnosis.**

Examination of thyroid status

1 Introduce yourself to the patient and wash your hands.

2 Perform a general survey.
- Observe the patient's demeanour. Are they anxious and fidgety, suggesting thyrotoxicosis, or are they slow and lethargic, suggesting hypothyroidism? Is the patient thin or fat?

3 Examine the hands for:
- fine tremor (place a piece of paper on the patient's outstretched arms, with the palms facing down and the fingers extended and separated)
- thyroid acropachy (a form of nail clubbing)
- onycholysis (separation of the nail from the nail bed)
- warm, moist, sweaty palms
- palmar erythema
- pulse (tachycardia, atrial fibrillation)
- vitiligo.

4 Check the eyes for:
- lid retraction (upper lid higher than normal, lower lid in correct position)
- lid lag – gently restrain the patient's head to prevent movement and ask the patient to follow your finger with their eyes as you lower it slowly from above. Do *not* do this in a rapid fashion. Lid lag occurs when the upper lid does not keep pace with the eyeball, and is due to spasm of the smooth muscle in the upper eyelid secondary to increased sympathetic tone in thyrotoxicosis
- proptosis/exophthalmos (look from in front, the side and from above; the sclera is visible below or all around the iris)
- chemosis
- ophthalmoplegia (eye movements)
- optic nerve involvement (visual acuity).

5 Thyroid gland examination.

6 Reflexes and pretibial myxoedema.

7 Ask the patient to stand up with their arms across their chest.
   ❱ Look for proximal myopathy, which can occur in
     hypothyroidism or hyperthyroidism.

8 Thank the patient and wash your hands.

9 Summarise and offer your differential diagnosis.

Assessment of thyroid status

Hyperthyroid	Hypothyroid
• General – restlessness, anxiety, weight loss, intolerance of heat	• General – dull, mental lethargy, intolerance of low temperatures, brittle hair
• Hands – nails (acropachy, onycholysis), palms (sweaty, warm, palmar erythema), fine tremor, pulse (tachycardic, AF)	• Hands – palms (dry, rough, inelastic, cold, pale), pulse (bradycardic), carpal tunnel (positive Tinel's sign)
• Eyes – lid lag, lid retraction, exophthalmos/proptosis, ophthalmoplegia, chemosis	• Eyes – periorbital puffiness, loss of outer one-third of eyebrows
• Neck – goitre, scars	• Neck – goitre, scars
• Reflexes – brisk	• Reflexes – delayed ankle jerks
• Legs and skin – pretibial myxoedema, vitiligo	

'Please ask this patient some questions . . .': thyroid status

Local pressure symptoms:
▶ neck lumps – duration, change in size with time, etc.
▶ pain
▶ dysphagia
▶ stridor/dyspnoea
▶ hoarseness
▶ cosmesis.

Questions about thyroid status:
▶ Are you on any medication?
▶ Have you had any thyroid operations, or radioiodine treatments, in the past?
▶ Do you prefer hot or cold conditions?
▶ Have you lost or gained weight?
▶ How are your bowels?
▶ How is your appetite?
▶ Do you get palpitations?
▶ Have your periods changed?
▶ Have you noticed any change in your appearance/face?
▶ Have you become more anxious?
▶ Has your skin/hair changed?
▶ Do you have any eye symptoms?

Common causes of neck swellings in the MRCS clinical exam

Midline neck swelling	Lateral neck swelling
• Sebaceous cyst	• Sebaceous cyst
• Lipoma	• Lipoma
• Thyroglossal cyst	• Cervical lymph node
• Solitary nodule of thyroid isthmus	• Thyroid gland enlargement
• Pyramidal thyroid lobe	• Branchial cyst
• Dermoid cyst	• Carotid body tumour
• Plunging ranula	• Pharyngeal pouch
• Pretracheal, prelaryngeal (level VI) lymph node	• Cystic hygroma

Causes of thyroid goitres

Simple goitres:

▶ physiological – pregnancy, puberty, lactation, menstruation
▶ pathological – iodine deficiency, goitrogens
▶ multinodular goitre.

Inflammatory:

▶ thyroiditis (Hashimoto's, de Quervain's, Riedel's).

Neoplastic:

▶ papillary
▶ follicular/Hurthle
▶ anaplastic
▶ medullary
▶ lymphoma.

Toxic:

▶ Graves
▶ solitary toxic adenoma/nodule
▶ multinodular goitre (Plummer's disease).

Rare: TB, amyloid, syphilis, HIV, lithium and sarcoid.

The solitary thyroid nodule

Differential diagnosis includes:

▶ adenoma/simple hyperplastic nodule
▶ simple thyroid cyst

- haemorrhage into a cyst/nodule
- prominent nodule in a multinodular goitre
- enlarged lobe (e.g. Hashimoto's thyroiditis)
- carcinoma – primary or rarely secondary.

The breast examination

1 **Introduce yourself to the patient and wash your hands.**
Position the patient at 45°.

Ensure that there is adequate privacy, comfort for the patient and exposure.

Alert the examiner to the fact that you would wish for a nurse chaperone to be present in a real-life clinical setting.

2 **General inspection.**
JACCOL (jaundice, anaemia, cyanosis, clubbing, oedema, lymphadenopathy), cachexia.

3 **Local inspection.**
Ask the patient to raise their arms slowly up into the air. Underlying disease often manifests as increased asymmetry during this manoeuvre.

Ask the patient to place their hands behind their head (look in the axilla, under the breasts in the inframammary fold).

Ask the patient to place their hands on their hips and press inward. This tenses the underlying pectoral muscles and has the effect of accentuating any differences between the breasts.

Ask the patient to lean forwards and/or lean back (this is helpful for demonstrating abnormalities in large pendulous breasts).

Look for:
‣ asymmetry
‣ nipple changes
‣ scars
‣ skin changes
‣ skin tethering and peau d'orange
‣ lumps and swellings
‣ late effects of radiotherapy
‣ lymphoedema.

Look specifically:
‣ at the inframammary fold, by lifting up each breast
‣ in the axilla for scars, swellings, and effects of radiotherapy
‣ at the back for evidence of latissimus dorsi reconstruction
‣ at the abdomen for evidence of TRAM flap reconstruction
‣ for the presence or absence of the pectoralis major muscle if

27

the patient has had a mastectomy (radical versus modified radical mastectomy), by asking the patient to press their hands against their hips.

4 **Palpation.**
Examine the unaffected breast first. Try to avoid calling it the 'normal' breast. Cover up the breast that is not being examined to preserve the patient's dignity. Then ask the patient to put their hand behind their head and roll slightly to the contralateral side. This makes the breast lie flat on the chest wall, providing a firm surface for palpation.

Ask about tenderness.

▶ Examine the six areas in each breast (four quadrants, axillary tail of Spence, and nipple–areolar complex).

▶ Mention that you would like to try to express discharge from the nipple by palpating the retro-areolar tissue (this is rarely requested to be performed in the clinical examination).

▶ Do not forget to palpate the inframammary fold.

If you find a lump, it is important to test for fixity to the underlying muscle by simultaneously asking the patient to press their hands into their hips to tense the underlying pectoralis major muscle while you palpate the breast lump.

▶ Define the characteristics of the lump, as you would for any other lump.

▶ Examine the contralateral breast (six areas).

▶ Examine both axillae for lymphadenopathy (note that the axilla has four walls and an apex). To examine the right axilla, support the patient's arm with your right arm and palpate with your left hand. To examine the left axilla, support the patient's left arm with your left arm and palpate with the fingertips of your right hand.

▶ Check for supraclavicular lymph nodes.

In the post-mastectomy breast, also test for surgical complications:

▶ sensation in the distribution of the intercostobrachial nerve (T2, sensation in armpit)

▶ winging of the scapula (long thoracic nerve damage, C5/6/7).

5 Finishing statement.

> *'To complete my examination I would like to examine the chest, back and abdomen (for hepatomegaly), and perform a full neurological examination.'*

You should complete a general physical examination to determine the patient's fitness for surgery.

6 Thank the patient and wash your hands.

7 Summarise and offer your differential diagnosis.

'Please ask this patient some questions . . .': breast

It is important to question the patient about the following:

- age of patient
- lump – rate of growth, changes with menstrual cycle
- nipple discharge – serous/serosanguinous/green/bloody/milk
- pain – cyclical/non-cyclical
- previous breast disease and treatments
- previous mammograms and results
- menstrual history – menarche, menopause, oral contraceptive pill use, hormone replacement therapy
- obstetric history – breastfeeding and complications, parity
- family history – breast, bowel or ovarian carcinoma (BRCA 1/2)
- radiation exposure (e.g. radiotherapy for Hodgkin's disease)
- symptoms of possible metastatic disease – other lumps (e.g. axilla), backache, breathlessness, headaches, tiredness, anorexia, weight loss, etc.

The musculoskeletal and neurological systems

'Please ask this patient some questions . . .': orthopaedics

Important questions to ask with regard to any joint include:
- age and occupation of the patient
- pain (including the presence of night pain and analgesic requirements)
- stiffness (including diurnal variation)
- swelling
- deformity
- instability
- neurological symptoms – changes in sensibility (numbness, tingling), weakness
- vascular symptoms – coldness and colour changes
- other joints affected
- history of trauma and previous treatments
- functional status – walking aids (sticks, crutches, frame), ability to get out of a chair, going to shops, walking a distance, use of stairs, getting in and out of car, putting on socks and shoes, getting in and out of bath
- impact on the patient's life (work, sleep, etc.)
- home circumstances – type of accommodation, stairs, rails, home help, etc.

For the upper limb, also ask about:
- hand dominance
- functional status – writing, feeding, washing, brushing hair, dressing, etc.

For the lower limb, also ask about:
- limping.

For the knee joint, also ask about:
- locking
- giving way.

For the back, also ask about:
- sphincter disturbances – bladder and bowels.

The hip examination

1 **Introduce yourself to the patient and wash your hands.**
   Start with the patient standing, and fully expose the hip joint,
   including the joint above and below it (back and knees).
      Ask about pain.
      The examination of the hip joint follows the same logical pat-
   tern as examination of any other joint. This includes the following
   elements:
   ▶ Look
   ▶ Feel
   ▶ Move
   ▶ Special tests

2 **Look (general).**
   ▶ Look around the patient's bed for walking aids, shoe raises,
     etc.
   ▶ Walk – assess the patient's gait.

3 **Look (specific).**
   ▶ Front – scars, wasting of quadriceps, sinuses, deformities.
     Put your hands on both ASIS to check whether they are level
     (assess for pelvic tilt).
   ▶ Sides – scars, wasting muscles, sinuses, exaggerated lordosis of
     the spine.
   ▶ Behind – scars, wasting glutei/hamstrings, tufts of hair,
     scoliosis, sinuses.

4 **Trendelenburg's test.**
   Demonstrate to the patient first:

   *'I'm now going to ask you to stand on one leg. When I ask you, can
   you please do it like this?'*

Ask the patient to stand on their good leg first, and then to stand
on their bad leg. Stand in front of the patient and provide support
to stop them falling over. We recommend that you perform the test
standing facing the patient and with the patient resting their hands
on your shoulders. Put your hands on their anterior superior
iliac spines to elicit pelvic tilt. If this is positive, the pelvis droops

opposite the bad hip and the patient lurches to the side of the problem. *Ideally you need to wait at least 30 seconds for the muscles to fatigue.* Alternatively, you can use the *indirect* method with their hands on your palms.

5 **Leg lengths.**

Ask the patient to lie supine with one pillow.

At this point, measure the leg lengths (apparent and true). It is helpful to ask the patient to *'Please lie straight in the bed like a soldier standing to attention.'*

▶ Measure the *apparent* leg length from the xiphisternum to the tip of the medial malleolus. The xiphisternum is more reliable as a proximal landmark than the umbilicus, as the site of the umbilicus may be affected by previous surgery. It may be easier to ask the patient to hold the proximal end of the tape measure for you on the xiphisternum.

▶ Measure the *true* leg length from the ASIS (which may be found easily by running your finger up the inguinal ligament) to the tip of the medial malleolus (run your finger up from the calcaneum to the inferior edge of the medial malleolus). You must square the pelvis and ensure that the patella and medial malleoli are together.

▶ Perform the *Galeazzi test* with the heels together. Look from the side and the end of the bed. Look to see if the shortening, if any, is in the femur (above the knee) or the tibia (below the knee). If you are unsure of the result of the test, flex both hips and knees to 90° and look at the knees from the side.

▶ Supratrochanteric leg length discrepancy is assessed using *Bryant's method.* Compare the distance between the ASIS and the greater trochanter on both sides.

6 **Feel** (ask about pain again before you continue).

▶ Temperature of the joint (assess with the back of the hand).

▶ Tenderness of the hip joint/head of femur. The hip joint lies deep to the femoral artery at the mid-inguinal point (halfway between the ASIS and the symphysis pubis). However, mention that the hip is deep and difficult to feel.

▶ Palpate the ischial tuberosity, greater trochanter and tendon of adductor longus.

▶ Feel for inguinal lymph nodes.

▶ Check for joint crepitus – with one hand over the hip joint, roll the femur laterally and medially.

▶ *Thomas's test*: Assess for a fixed flexion deformity (FFD) of the hip joint. Place your hand under the lumbar lordosis and flex the patient's good hip (ask the patient to bring their good knee up towards their chest and hold it there). This obliterates the lumbar lordosis. Then exclude an FFD of the bad hip by observing its lift off the bed, and assess flexion of the good hip. Keep your hand under the lumbar region throughout and then flex the bad hip to exclude an FFD of the good hip. *Note: You must watch the patient's face for signs of discomfort when extending the hip from the flexed position.* Summarise your findings aloud – for example, flexion of good hip from 0 to 120°, flexion of bad hip from 20 to 120°, implying an FFD of the bad hip of 20°.

7 Move.

▶ Hip flexion has already been assessed in Thomas's test.

▶ Test internal/external rotation in extension, looking at the rotation of the patellae to assess the degree of movement. Assess the range of movement and note any crepitus.

▶ Test internal/external rotation in 90° of flexion. Assess the range of movement and note any crepitus.

▶ Test for abduction/adduction of the hip, while placing your fingers on the contralateral ASIS to fix the pelvis (you could also hang the contralateral leg off the side of the bed to lock/fix the pelvis). The end point should be when the pelvis starts to move. You may need to go around the bed to test for hip abduction on the contralateral side. Assess the range of movement and note any crepitus.

8 Complete the examination.

▶ Turn the patient prone and formerly assess extension (although this is of limited use if Thomas's test is positive).

▶ Check the neurovascular status.

▶ Examine the joint above and below (back/knee).

▶ Assess the impact of the joint condition on the patient's life.

▶ Request an X-ray of the hip joint.

▶ Assess the patient's fitness for surgery.

9 Thank the patient and wash your hands.

10 Summarise and offer your differential diagnosis.

The Trendelenburg test explained

This question is a favourite of examiners, so it is worth spending a moment discussing it. Put simply, the test is an assessment of insufficiency of the hip abductor system.

Ask the patient to stand on their good leg and flex the other leg at the knee. The opposite side of the pelvis should rise to help to balance the trunk on the leg by bringing the centre of gravity over the weight-bearing foot. This involves the use of the hip abductors – the gluteus medius and minimus.

This manoeuvre is then repeated by asking the patient to stand on their bad leg. The test is positive if the opposite side of the pelvis falls and the patient has difficulty standing. You may notice that the patient throws the upper part of their body over the affected hip in order to compensate for the loss of balance due to the pelvic dip on the contralateral side (*Trendelenburg lurch*).

A Trendelenburg test can be positive for two main reasons – neurological or mechanical. *Neurological* causes can be due to generalised motor weakness as seen with myelomeningocele and spinal cord lesions, or more specific problems, such as superior gluteal nerve dysfunction/injury (e.g. following hip surgery). The *mechanical* causes include conditions that affect the abductor muscle lever arm, such as:

▶ congenital dislocation of the hip
▶ coxa vara
▶ fractures of the femoral neck
▶ dislocation or subluxation of the hip joint
▶ neuromuscular diseases (e.g. poliomyelitis)
▶ pain arising in the hip joint, inhibiting the gluteal muscles.

These conditions shorten the length of the muscle from its origin to its insertion, and significantly reduce its strength.

It should be noted that the test is not valid in children below the age of 4 years, and that it has a 10% false-positive rate due to pain, generalised weakness, poor cooperation or bad balance.

The knee examination

1 **Introduce yourself to the patient and wash your hands.**
   Position – start with the patient standing, obtain full exposure of the knee joint so that you can visualise the joint above and below, and ask the patient to remove their socks.
   Ask about pain.

2 **Look (general).**
   ▶ Around the bed for walking aids, shoe raises, etc.
   ▶ Watch the patient walk.
   ▶ Watch the patient squat.
   ▶ Inspect the patient from in front with the legs together – look for scars, wasting of quadriceps muscle (especially vastus medialis), sinuses, FFD/deformities, valgus/varus deformities (alignment).
   ▶ Inspect from the side – look for scars, wasting muscles, sinuses, FFD.
   ▶ Inspect from behind – look for scars, popliteal swellings.

3 **Look (specific).**
   Lie the patient down (ideally flat on the bed to relax the hamstrings, but 45° is permissible). Stand on the same side as the knee you have been asked to examine.
   ▶ Inspect briefly again – look for any swellings of the suprapatellar pouch for an effusion.
   ▶ Look carefully for arthroscopic scars either side of the patellar tendon, anteromedially and anterolaterally.
   ▶ Measure the leg circumference 15 cm above the tibial tubercle for quadriceps wasting.
   ▶ Ask the patient to push their heels down into the bed and feel the bulk of the quadriceps muscle. To exclude an FFD, put your hand underneath the popliteal fossa. If an FFD is present, put one hand on the patella and one hand on the quadriceps and try to straighten the knee to confirm that it is fixed.

4 **Feel.**
   ▶ Temperature of joint (assess with the back of the hand).
   ▶ Test for a joint effusion:
   — For a small effusion, perform the *sweep test*. Empty the

medial side of the knee joint by sweeping the back of your hand up the medial side of the knee, then sweep your hand down the lateral side. As the fluid returns, the dimple on the medial side of the knee pops out.

— For a moderate effusion, perform the *patellar tap test*. With your thumb and two fingers press down on the patella.

— For a large effusion, try to ballott the fluid between the medial and lateral aspects of the joint (*cross-fluctuation test*).

▶ Flex the patient's knee to 45° and palpate the joint (remember to palpate the medial tibial condyle, medial joint line, medial femoral condyle, medial collateral ligament, tibial tuberosity, patellar tendon, upper and lower poles of the patella, round the back in the popliteal fossa, lateral femoral condyle, lateral joint line, lateral tibial condyle, lateral collateral ligament, and head of the fibula). As you palpate, remember to look at the patient's face for signs of discomfort.

▶ Straighten the knee and try to move the patella in two planes (assess for patellofemoral joint crepitus and tenderness). Palpate along the extensor mechanism for any gaps or defects.

5 Move.

▶ Ask the patient to point their toes to the ceiling, perform a straight leg raise and then lower the leg back down again (assess the extensor mechanism and look for an 'extensor lag').

▶ Check for passive hyperextension (genu recurvatum) by placing one hand on the patella and lifting up the heel.

▶ Ask the patient to bring their heel into their bottom as far as possible (active flexion).

▶ Test for passive flexion and feel for crepitus with your hand on the patella (you can also screen the hip joint at this point by testing internal/external rotation at the hip joint, remembering that hip pathology can refer pain to the knee).

▶ Grade the power of knee flexion and extension from 1 to 5 (MRC Scale).

6 Special tests/ligaments.

▶ Ask the patient to put their heels together, with the knees flexed to 45°, and look for a *posterior sag*, which is indicative of a posterior cruciate ligament tear. The importance of a posterior sag is that, if present, it can lead to a false-positive anterior drawer test (i.e. the tibia can be pulled forwards to a neutral position). Therefore always look for a posterior sag first before performing the anterior drawer test.

▶ Perform the *drawer test* to check the cruciate ligaments. This can be performed by placing your elbow on the patient's feet, or you may prefer to sit by the patient's feet. If the latter technique is used, be careful not to hurt the patient. Either way, *don't forget to disengage the hamstrings!* Pull the tibia forwards (anterior drawer) to test the anterior cruciate ligament. Push the tibia firmly backwards (posterior drawer) to test the posterior cruciate ligament.

▶ Perform *Lachman's test*. This is most easily performed by placing your knee under the patient's knee that is being examined. Hold the distal femur down and pull the tibia upwards to stress the anterior cruciate ligament.

▶ Test the collateral ligaments of the knee joint in extension and slight flexion with *valgus/varus stress*.

▶ Test the menisci by performing *McMurray's test*. Flex and externally rotate the knee and then slowly extend the knee to stress the medial meniscus. Flex and internally rotate the knee and then slowly extend the knee to stress the lateral meniscus. A palpable click and/or pain during the test are suggestive of a tear.

▶ Screen for hip pathology by checking internal and external rotation of the hip joint in extension and flexion.

7 **Complete the examination.**
Check the patient's neurovascular status:
▶ the distal pulses
▶ sensation – L4 medial malleolus, L5 hallux (medial aspect), S1 foot (lateral aspect).

Offer an examination of the joints above and below (hip, back and ankle joints), and request a weight-bearing X-ray of the knee joint.

8 **Thank the patient and wash your hands.**

9 **Summarise and offer your differential diagnosis.**

The shoulder examination

1 **Introduce yourself to the patient and wash your hands.**
Stand the patient up and obtain adequate exposure (including the joint above and below).
Ask about pain.

2 **Look.**
  ▶ Around the bed.
  ▶ Inspect from in front – scars (arthroscopic scars may be found front and back), sinuses, contour of the shoulder/squaring off, muscle wasting of deltoid, trapezius.
  ▶ Inspect from the side – scars.
  ▶ Inspect the back of the joint – scars, contour, wasting of supraspinatus/ infraspinatus.
  ▶ Ask the patient to push with both hands against a wall, and look for winging of the scapula (serratus anterior, long thoracic nerve of Bell, C5/6/7).

3 **Feel.**
  ▶ Temperature.
  ▶ Sternoclavicular joint, along the clavicle, supraclavicular fossa, coracoid process, acromion/acromioclavicular joint (ACJ), subacromial space. Abduct the humerus and feel the glenohumeral joint line.
  ▶ Axilla (for osteomas, lipomas, lymph nodes, etc.).
  ▶ Greater tuberosity of humerus, bicipital groove, spine of scapula, inferior pole of scapula, supraspinatus and infraspinatus, medial border scapula, cervical spine.

4 **Move** (active before passive).
It may help to demonstrate the movement first and then ask the patient to follow you. During passive movements, check for crepitus.
  ▶ Abduction – ask the patient to raise both hands above their head. Look for a 'painful arc.'
  ▶ Adduction – ask the patient to bring their arm over to the opposite shoulder (assess for OA of the ACJ at this point – *Scarf test*).
  ▶ Forward flexion.
  ▶ Extension.
  ▶ External rotation – first with the elbows flexed to 90°, and then ask the patient to place their hands behind their head.

- Internal rotation – ask the patient to place their hands as far up behind their back as possible (normally one should be able to get up as high as the sixth thoracic vertebra).
- Circumduction.

5 **Special tests.**
'*I would now like to test the individual muscles of the* **rotator cuff.**'
Grade the power of each from 1 to 5 (MRC Scale).
- *Supraspinatus* – thumbs down test/Jobe's test/empty can test.
- *Teres minor* and *infraspinatus* – resisted external rotation.
- *Subscapularis* – Gerber's lift-off test, or Napoleon's belly-press test (as in Gerber's lift-off test, push posteriorly).

'*I would now like to test for* **impingement.**'
- Neer's sign and test – with the patient's thumb down, put one hand on their shoulder and with your other hand passively lift up their hand in the plane of the scapula (forward flexion) until they experience pain. Pain during this manoeuvre is a positive *Neer's sign*, and pain abolished with local anaesthetic infiltration is a positive *Neer's test*.
- Hawkins' test – raise the patient's arm to 90° forward flexion and bend the elbow to 90°. Then passively internally rotate the shoulder (i.e. thumb pointed down). Pain is indicative of impingement.

'*I would now like to test for a* **ruptured long head of biceps.**'
Test for a 'biceps bulge' by flexing the elbow against resistance.

'*I would now like to test the* **axillary nerve.**'
Test sensation in the regimental badge area.

6 **Complete the examination.**
- Check the neurovascular status.
- Examine the neck and elbow.
- Request an X-ray of the shoulder joint.

7 **Thank the patient and wash your hands.**

8 **Summarise and offer your differential diagnosis.**

The elbow examination

1 **Introduce yourself to the patient and wash your hands.**
   Fully expose the joint above and below the elbow.
      Ask about pain.

2 **Look.**
   Inspect the front, the side and the back of the joint.
   ▶ Skin – for scars, bruising, sinuses, psoriatic plaques.
   ▶ Soft tissues – for muscle wasting, swellings, rheumatoid nodules, olecranon bursitis, gouty tophi.
   ▶ Bone – for deformities (cubitus valgus, varus).

3 **Feel.**
   ▶ Medial epicondyle.
   ▶ Lateral epicondyle.
   ▶ Olecranon.
   ▶ Head of the radius and ulna.
   ▶ Over the ulnar nerve (behind the medial epicondyle).
   ▶ Intercondylar line.
   ▶ Joint line (loose bodies).
   ▶ Antecubital fossa (tendon biceps brachii, brachial artery, median nerve).

4 **Move.**
   ▶ Assess flexion and extension at the elbow joint (this is best illustrated to the examiners by asking the patient to put their arms out to the side, i.e. abducting at the shoulder to 90° and then asking the patient to flex/extend at the elbow joint).
   ▶ Test supination and pronation with the elbows flexed at the sides.

5 **Special tests.**
   ▶ Stress the *collateral ligaments*.
   ▶ Reproduction of paraesthesia on tapping over the ulnar nerve behind the medial epicondyle (Tinel's sign).
   ▶ Elbow flexion test for ulnar nerve entrapment (cubital tunnel syndrome).
   ▶ Special test for tennis elbow (lateral epicondylitis) – actively extend the wrist against resistance (Thomsen's test).

6 **Complete the examination.**
   ▶ Check the neurovascular status.
   ▶ Offer an examination of the joint above and below.
   ▶ Request an X-ray of the elbow joint.

7 **Thank the patient and wash your hands.**

8 **Summarise and offer your differential diagnosis.**

Examination of the foot and ankle

1 **Introduce yourself to the patient and wash your hands.**
Fully expose the leg up to the thigh.
Ask about pain.

2 **Look.**
- Around the bed for shoes and walking aids.
- Examine the patient's shoes for wear and tear.
- Watch the patient walk (e.g. foot drop secondary to nerve injury at fibula).
- Watch the patient walk 'heel-to-toes.'
- Watch the patient walk on tiptoe (plantar flexion of foot; S1, 2).
- Watch the patient walk on their heels (dorsiflexion of foot; L4, 5).
- Ask the patient to stand on tiptoe on both feet. Look from behind for normal varus/inversion of the hindfoot.
- Ask the patient to stand on tiptoe on one foot.
- Ask the patient to stand with one foot in front of the other. Look at the ankle and the front, sides and back of the foot to assess the integrity of the three arches (medial, lateral and transverse), the 'too many toes' sign (a sign of dysfunction of the tibialis posterior tendon), deformities, muscle wasting, etc.
- Look at the nails, the toes and the soles of the feet.
- Look in between the toes (corns, callosities, ulcers, etc.).

3 **Feel.**
Ask the patient to sit on a chair.
- Temperature.
- Capillary refill.
- Achilles tendon (feel for a defect).
- Lateral/medial malleoli and ankle joint line.
- Peroneal tendons behind the lateral malleolus.
- Medial/lateral ligaments of ankle and extensor tendons.
- The foot bones – os calcis, tarsal bones and metatarsals.
- Squeeze metatarsophalangeal joints 1 to 5 to assess for tenderness (RA), and test for subluxation of MTP joints.
- Plantar surface – plantar fascia, heel, head of fifth metatarsal, callus/callosities, Morton's neuroma.

▶ Pulses (posterior tibial, dorsalis pedis).

4 Move.
▶ Dorsiflexion/plantarflexion of the ankle joint (Apley's test).
▶ Subtalar joint (inversion/eversion).
▶ Mid-tarsal joint (supination/pronation, abduction/adduction).
▶ Metatarsophalangeal, interphalangeal joints (flexion/extension). Ask the patient to curl their toes and then extend them.
▶ Inversion and eversion against resistance (palpate the tendons of the tibialis posterior and peronei tendons as you do this).

5 Special tests.
▶ *Simmond's/Thompson's test* (tendo Achilles rupture).
▶ *Grind test* to check for hallux rigidus.
▶ *Mulder's click/sign* for Morton's neuroma.
▶ *Anterior drawer test* – for joint instability.
▶ *Tinel's test* – percuss over the posterior tibial nerve (tarsal tunnel syndrome).

6 Complete the examination.
▶ Check the neurovascular status.
▶ Offer an examination of the knee joint, hip and back.
▶ Request a joint X-ray.

7 Thank the patient and wash your hands.

8 Summarise and offer your differential diagnosis.

Examination of the hands

1 **Introduce yourself to the patient and wash your hands.**
   Obtain adequate exposure up to and including the elbows, bearing in mind that the elbow is the origin of the long flexor/extensor tendons. The presence of rheumatoid nodules at the elbow is a vital clue!

   Ask for a pillow and place both hands on the pillow, dorsum side up.

   Ask whether there is any tenderness.

2 **Look, Look, Look.**
   The most important part of the examination of the hands is inspection. This will guide you on how to proceed. If there is something obvious, go for it and describe the features of the lump, etc. (e.g. rheumatoid nodule). For example, in the case of rheumatoid arthritis, say something like:

   > *'There is a bilateral and symmetrical polyarthropathy affecting the small joints of the hand . . . with sparing of the DIPJs and involvement of the MCPJs/PIPJs.'*

   If there is nothing obvious on inspection, the station is likely to represent a rheumatological, orthopaedic, neurological or vascular case. Proceed as follows – and above all be systematic!
   - Skin – nail changes (pitting, vasculitic changes), spindling of fingers, fusiform swellings, bruising, purpura, thinning of the skin, psoriatic plaques, gouty tophi, SCARS (e.g. a dorsal wrist scar implies previous synovectomy, or arthrodesis in RA, whereas a scar over the head of the ulna implies a previous Darrach procedure). If there is any soft tissue swelling visible, mention that you will not know whether it is bony or inflammatory until you palpate it.
   - Muscles – wasting, dorsal guttering, look specifically for wasting of the first dorsal interosseous.
   - Bones – with the hand at rest, the fingers should be held in a normal cascade. Look for deformities (ulnar deviation of fingers, Swan-neck deformities, Boutonnière deformities, subluxation at MCPJs, radial deviation and volar subluxation at the wrist joint, caput ulnae, Z-shaped thumb, Heberden's

nodes, Bouchard's nodes, squaring off of the thumb, involvement/sparing DIPJs).
▶ Watch the patient lift their hands off the pillow and look for a dropped finger/thumb (evidence of extensor tendon rupture) and wrist drop.

Ask the patient to turn their hands over so that you can view the volar/palmar surface (comment on the range of movement, i.e. supination/pronation which principally takes place at the distal radio-ulnar joint). Comment on the volar/palmar surface as follows:
▶ Skin – look carefully for carpal tunnel scars which may be faint, pallor in the palmar creases, and palmar erythema.
▶ Muscles – wasting of the thenar and hypothenar eminences.
▶ Bones – in particular, are any fingers held in an attitude of flexion? (Avoid the term FFD at this stage, as you won't know if it is fixed until you feel).

Ask the patient to put their hands behind their head, and then check the elbows for:
▶ scars around the medial epicondyle/ulnar nerve
▶ rheumatoid nodules
▶ psoriatic plaques
▶ gouty tophi.

Do not forget to inspect the ulnar aspect of the wrist, which is easily missed.

3 **Feel.**
   ▶ Temperature.
   ▶ Capillary refill, pulses (with or without Allen's test).
   ▶ Squeeze the metacarpals together and assess for tenderness.
   ▶ Feel each joint in turn to determine the levels affected in the hand and whether active inflammation or inactive disease is present.
   ▶ Feel rheumatoid nodules, synovitis, bony nodules, nodularity of Dupuytren's disease, nodules along flexor tendons/A1 pulley in trigger finger.

4 **Move.**
Ask the patient to perform the following movements:
▶ Make a fist (can they bury the fingers?).
▶ Squeeze your fingers, to assess power.
▶ Flex one finger at a time, to touch the thenar eminence.
▶ Spread their fingers wide apart.
▶ Demonstrate playing the piano with their fingers.
▶ Oppose thumb to each finger.
▶ Place their hands in a 'pray position' (wrist extension).
▶ Place their hands in a 'reverse pray position' (wrist flexion).
▶ Wrap fingers around the wrist.
▶ Circumduct the wrist joint.

5 **Nerve function** (see later chapters).
▶ Radial nerve.
▶ Median nerve.
▶ Ulnar nerve.

6 **Tendons** (see later chapters).
▶ Flexor digitorum profundus and superficialis.
▶ Extensor and flexor pollicis longus.
▶ The long extensors.

7 **Functional status.** Ask the patient to:
▶ write
▶ pick up a coin from the pillow
▶ unfasten and refasten a garment button
▶ pretend to use a key.

8 **Special tests.**
Finkelstein's test (De Quervain's tenovaginitis stenosans).

9 **Complete the examination.**
▶ Ask the patient some questions to investigate the effects of the condition on their life.
▶ Check the neurovascular status.
▶ Assess the functional status.
▶ Request X-rays.
▶ Offer to examine other joints and look for extra-articular manifestations of rheumatoid disease (eyes, chest, skin, heart, abdomen, neurological, etc.).

10 Thank the patient and wash your hands.

11 Summarise and offer your differential diagnosis.

Examination of the thumb

1 **Introduce yourself to the patient and wash your hands.**
Obtain adequate exposure up to and including the elbows. The presence of rheumatoid nodules at the elbow is a vital clue!
Ask about pain.

2 **Look.**
- Nail changes.
- Muscle wasting.
- Heberden's nodes, Bouchard's nodules (OA).
- Z-thumb (RA).

3 **Feel.**
- Scaphoid.
- Metacarpal.
- Proximal phalanx.
- Distal phalanx.
- Tendons surrounding the anatomical snuffbox.
- Nodules (trigger thumb).
- Along the joint lines for tenderness.
- Test sensation at the thumb tip and along the sides (median nerve, digital branches).

4 **Move.**
- Extend the thumb.
- Flex the thumb across the palm.
- Adduct.
- Abduct (perform the 'pen test'; *see* 'Approach to the median nerve palsy', page 55).
- Opposition to each finger in turn.
- Retropulsion test (*see* 'Approach to the radial nerve palsy', page 58).
- DIPJ flexion (FPL tendon).
- 'OK' sign test (tests FPL thumb, FDP index finger) (*see* Figure 1).
- Circumduction.

5 **Special tests.**
- Test ligaments (gamekeeper's thumb).

- ▶ *Froment's test* (*see* 'Approach to the ulnar nerve palsy', page 53).
- ▶ *Finkelstein's test* (De Quervain's tenosynovitis).
- ▶ *Grind test* (carpometacarpal OA).
- ▶ *Allen's test* and capillary refill.

6 **Functional status.** Ask the patient to:
- ▶ make a fist
- ▶ pick up a coin
- ▶ grip a key
- ▶ unfasten and refasten a garment button
- ▶ write with a pen.

7 **Complete the examination.**
- ▶ Ask the patient some questions to investigate the effects of the condition on their life.
- ▶ Check the neurovascular status.
- ▶ Request X-rays.

8 **Thank the patient and wash your hands.**

9 **Summarise and offer your differential diagnosis.**

Approach to the ulnar nerve palsy

1 **Introduce yourself to the patient and wash your hands.**
The patient's sleeves must be rolled up to obtain full exposure.
Ask about pain.

2 **Look (dorsum surface).**
   ▶ Skin – pulp atrophy, scars, cigarette burns, brittle nails.
   ▶ Muscle – wasting of first dorsal web space/interosseous, dorsal guttering.
   ▶ Bone – clawing (ulnar paradox).

3 **Look (palmar surface).**
Skin – as above.
   ▶ Muscle – wasting of hypothenar eminence, wasting of medial forearm muscles.
   ▶ Bone – ask the patient to lay their hand flat on the table so that you can assess whether or not any flexion deformity is fixed ('table-top test').

Ask the patient to place their hands behind their head. Then check the elbows for scars around the medial epicondyle/forearm/wrist, and check the elbow for cubitus valgus (tardy ulnar syndrome).

4 **Feel.**
   ▶ Palpate along the ulnar nerve behind the medial epicondyle and at the wrist joint.
   ▶ Test the sensation over the tip of the little finger – volar surface (ask the patient to close their eyes and compare one hand/side with the other).
   ▶ Turn the hands over and test the dorsal cutaneous branch of the ulnar nerve (given off proximal to the wrist).

5 **Move.**
Test the muscles:
   ▶ First dorsal interosseous – resisted abduction of index finger and feel first dorsal web space.
   ▶ Abductor digiti minimi – do the same with the little finger.
   ▶ Hold a piece of paper in between the patient's fingers and ask them to try to stop you from pulling the paper out (this tests the finger adductors, i.e. palmar interossei).

- Ask the patient to spread their fingers apart and stop you from pushing them together (this tests the finger abductors, i.e. dorsal interossei).
- Ask the patient to put their hands together with the palms up and little fingers touching. Ask them to push the little fingers together (this tests the finger abductors).
- *Froment's test* for adductor pollicis – in ulnar nerve palsy, the flexor pollicis longus flexes the IPJ to compensate.
- Ulnar half of the FDP – bend the tip of the little finger at the DIPJ.
- Make a fist (grip hard and flex the wrist) – look for contraction of the FCU and the ulnar half of the FDP.
- To test the FCU, ask the patient to flex and adduct the wrist/ gripped hand against resistance (flexion and ulnar deviation at the wrist). Also with paralysis of the FCU, flexion at the wrist joint will result in abduction.
- Cross and reverse-cross the index and middle finger (this tests the interossei). Also known as the 'making a wish' sign, the patient will be unable to cross their index finger over the middle finger and vice versa, due to weakness of the intrinsics.

6 **Functional status.**

7 **Special tests.**
- *Tinel's percussion test* over Guyon's canal and at the elbow.
- *Elbow flexion test* (the patient flexes both elbows and holds them in close to the body. Wait 1 minute to see whether the patient develops paraesthesia).

8 **Complete the examination.**
- Ask the patient some questions to investigate the effect of the condition on their life.
- Examine the neck.
- Check the vascular status.
- Offer to arrange nerve conduction studies.

9 **Thank the patient and wash your hands.**

10 **Summarise and offer your differential diagnosis.**

Approach to the median nerve palsy

1 **Introduce yourself to the patient and wash your hands.**
    The patient's sleeves must be rolled up to obtain full exposure.
    Ask about pain.

2 **Look.**
    ▶ Skin – carpal tunnel scars (look on both sides – they may be faint), pulp atrophy, cigarette burns.
    ▶ Muscle – wasting of the thenar eminence, wasting of the lateral forearm flexors.
    ▶ Bone – simian thumb.
    ▶ Ask the patient to place their hands behind their head, and then check the elbows for cubitus valgus/varus from previous injuries, and scars around the elbow, forearm and wrist.

3 **Feel.**
    ▶ Test sensation over the tip of the index finger and over the thenar eminence (compare the two sides). Note that in carpal tunnel syndrome there is 'thenar sparing' as the palmar cutaneous branch is given off proximal to the flexor retinaculum.
    ▶ Feel for the median nerve where it is superficial at the wrist.

4 **Move.**
    Test the muscles (remember that the median nerve supplies the LOAF muscles in the hand, i.e. the lateral two lumbricals, opponens pollicis, abductor pollicis brevis and flexor pollicis brevis):
    ▶ Abductor pollicis brevis – the *pen-touching test*. Ask the patient to place the dorsum of their hand flat on a table and either to point their thumb towards the ceiling, or to touch your pen which is held directly above. Ask them to resist you pushing their thumb down. Look and feel simultaneously for muscle contraction in the thenar eminence.
    ▶ Opposition (thumb to each finger).
    ▶ '*OK*' *sign test* (this tests FPL thumb, FDP index finger, anterior interosseous branch of median nerve). If the FPL and FDP to the index are intact and working, the patient should be able to make an 'O' (tip-to-tip pinch). If not, only the pulps of the finger and thumb can be approximated, rather than the tips. To

test the strength of the muscles, try to break the circle between thumb and index finger (*see* Figure 1).

▶ Flexor pollicis longus – hold the base of the thumb and ask the patient to bend the tip of the thumb.

▶ Test the FDP – fix the PIPJ and isolate the DIPJ. Then ask the patient to bend the tip of the finger.

▶ Test the FDS – hold the other fingers down in extension to eliminate the FDP, and then ask the patient to flex the finger.

▶ Ask the patient to make a fist (look for the 'benediction sign'), and inspect the volar forearm for contraction of the palmaris longus and flexor carpi radialis (make a tight fist and flex at the wrist to contract the forearm muscles well).

▶ Ask the patient to flex at the wrist, and then look for ulnar deviation/adduction (unopposed action of the FCU because of weak forearm flexors).

▶ Finally, test the pronator teres (extend the elbow and pronate against resistance – test this as if to shake the patient's hand, and ask them to push against you).

5 **Functional status.**

6 **Special tests.**
▶ *Ochsner's clasp test.*
▶ *Tinel's sign* (tap over the median nerve from the top of the forearm down to the centre of the palm).
▶ *Phalen's test* (allow the wrists to fall freely into maximum flexion, and maintain the position for 60 seconds or more).
▶ *Durkan's test.*
▶ *Sphygmomanometer test.*

7 **Complete the examination.**
▶ Ask the patient some questions to investigate the effect of the condition on their life.
▶ Examine the patient's neck.
▶ Check the vascular status.
▶ Offer to arrange nerve conduction studies.
▶ Request an X-ray of the cervical spine, and consider an MRI of the neck.

8 **Thank the patient and wash your hands.**

9 Summarise and offer your differential diagnosis.

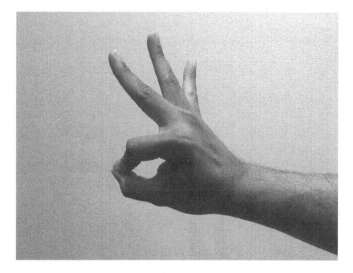

Figure 1: The 'OK' sign test: Pincer grip (median nerve); Finger abduction (ulnar nerve); Wrist dorsiflexion (radial nerve).

Approach to the radial nerve palsy

1 **Introduce yourself to the patient and wash your hands.**
   The patient's sleeves must be rolled up to obtain full exposure.
   Ask about pain.

2 **Look.**
   Dorsal and palmar surfaces.
   ▶ Skin – pulp atrophy, scars, cigarette burns.
   ▶ Muscle – wasting of the forearm extensors.
   ▶ Bone – wrist drop.
   ▶ Ask the patient to place their hands behind their head, and
     then check the elbows for scars (head radius fracture) and
     wasting of triceps.
   ▶ Ask the patient to lift their hand off the pillow, and then look
     for wrist drop.

3 **Feel.**
   ▶ Test sensation over the first dorsal web space (compare the two
     sides).
   ▶ Test sensation over the back of the forearm.

4 **Move.**
   Test the muscles:
   ▶ Test extension of the triceps muscle (for very high lesions).
   ▶ Test the brachioradialis (flex the elbow in mid-prone position
     against resistance).
   ▶ Test the supinator (elbow extended and supinate against
     resistance – test this by gripping the patient's hand with your
     opposite hand, i.e. grip their right hand with your left hand,
     and grip their left hand with your right hand). Ask them to
     push against you.
   ▶ Ask the patient to cock their wrist back against resistance
     (extensors of wrist joint).
   ▶ Test the extensors of the fingers (ask the patient to keep their
     fingers straight and stop you bending their fingers).
   ▶ Examine EPL by performing the *retropulsion test* (ask the
     patient to put their hand on a table, palm side down, and lift
     their thumb into the air, against resistance).

5 Functional status.

6 Complete the examination.
  ▶ Ask the patient some questions to investigate the effects of the condition on their life.
  ▶ Examine the patient's neck.
  ▶ Check the vascular status.
  ▶ Request an X-ray (look for fracture of the humerus).
  ▶ Offer to arrange nerve conduction studies.

7 Thank the patient and wash your hands.

8 Summarise and offer your differential diagnosis.

The back examination

1 **Introduce yourself to the patient and wash your hands.**
   Obtain adequate exposure.
   Ask about pain.

2 **Look.**
   ▶ Ask the patient to walk so that you can assess *gait*.
   ▶ Watch the patient walk on tiptoe (plantarflexion; S1,2).
   ▶ Watch the patient walk on their heels (dorsiflexion; L4,5).
   ▶ Skin – scars, sinuses, hairy tufts, café-au-lait spots.
   ▶ Soft tissues – muscle wasting.
   ▶ Bone – deformities to include scoliosis, kyphosis, lordosis, gibbus.
   ▶ Ask the patient to sit down or touch their toes, to exclude compensatory/postural scoliosis.

3 **Feel.**
   ▶ Palpate down from the cervical vertebrae, checking for step deformities and areas of tenderness.
   ▶ Palpate the sacroiliac joints on either side.
   ▶ Check for muscle spasm.
   ▶ Percuss down the midline and either side for tenderness.

4 **Move.**
   ▶ Forward flexion – ask the patient to touch their toes (if this is reduced, perform *Schober's test*). The patient should be able to reach within 7 cm of the floor.
   ▶ Extension – ask the patient to bend backwards.
   ▶ Lateral flexion – ask the patient to slide their hand down the side of each leg.
   ▶ Rotation – ask the patient to sit down, cross their arms across their body and twist to the other side.

   Lie the patient down on the couch.
   ▶ Screen the hip joint by testing internal/external rotation of the hip in 90° of flexion.
   ▶ Perform the *straight leg raise test (Lasègue's test)* and record the angle (in degrees).
   ▶ Perform the *sciatic nerve stretch test* (passive dorsiflexion of the foot; Bragard's sign).

▶ Consider the *femoral nerve stretch test* with the patient prone (*reverse Lasègue's test*).
▶ Test sensation in the dermatomes.
▶ Test extension of the hallux on each side (L5).
▶ Test the reflexes (ankle/knee).

5 **Special tests.**
   ▶ *Modified Schober's test* (mark the level between the iliac crests and 10 cm above, and then ask the patient to touch their toes. There should be more than a 5 cm increase in separation).
   ▶ *Heel–hips–occiput test* – also known as the *wall test* (AS).
   ▶ *Patrick's test* for SIJ (also known as the *Faber test*) and other SIJ tests.

6 **Complete the examination.**
   ▶ Check the neurovascular status (full neurological examination of the legs; assess the femoral pulses, as vascular and neurogenic claudication can mimic one another).
   ▶ Abdominal examination (e.g. AAA).
   ▶ Perform a digital rectal examination and check anal tone.
   ▶ Examine the hip joint.
   ▶ Request an ESR.
   ▶ Request X-rays of the cervical/thoracic/lumbar spine (AP and lateral). Also consider requesting an MRI of the spine.

7 **Thank the patient and wash your hands.**

8 **Summarise and offer your differential diagnosis.**

Upper limb neurology

1 **Introduce yourself to the patient and wash your hands.**
   Expose the upper body with the patient sitting or standing.
   Ask about pain.

2 **Look.**
   ▶ Around the bed for splints, collars, etc.
   ▶ Scars – neck, arms.
   ▶ Deformities.
   ▶ Muscle bulk – wasting.
   ▶ Tremors/fasciculations.
   ▶ Joints – swollen, erythematous.

3 **Feel.**
   ▶ Tone – rotate hands at wrist joints.
   ▶ Sensation:
     — *snuffbox* – radial nerve
     — *little finger* – ulnar nerve
     — *index finger* – median nerve.
   ▶ Offer to test other sensory modalities (vibration, joint position sense, pain, temperature, etc.).

4 **Move.**
   ▶ Power (compare both sides):
     — deltoids – try to push down elbows from a fixed abducted 'chicken-wing' position (C5,6)
     — biceps – try to extend flexed elbows (C5,6)
     — triceps – try to flex extended elbows (C7,8)
     — screening ulnar, median and radial nerves – 'OK' sign (*see* Figure 1)
     — wrist extension – try to push down dorsiflexed fists (radial nerve)
     — finger abduction – try to push in fingers held spread (ulnar nerve)
     — thumb abduction – try to push down upward-pointing thumbs (median nerve).
   ▶ Coordination:
     — finger to nose
     — alternating palm and dorsum claps.

▶ Reflexes:
  — biceps – (C5/6, musculocutaneous nerve)
  — supinator – (C6, radial nerve)
  — triceps – (C7/8, radial nerve).

5 **Special tests.**
  ▶ *Froment's test* – try to pull a piece of paper out from between the patient's thumb and palm. In ulnar nerve palsy, the flexor pollicis longus flexes the thumb IPJ to compensate for a paralysed adductor pollicis.
  ▶ *Phalen's test/Tinel tap* – carpal tunnel syndrome (median nerve).

6 **Thank the patient and wash your hands.**

7 **Summarise and offer your differential diagnosis.**

Lower limb neurology

1 **Introduce yourself to the patient and wash your hands.**
    Expose the lower limbs, with the patient in a standing position.
    Ask about pain.

2 **Look.**
    ▶ Around the bed for splints, walking aids, prostheses, orthoses,
        spinal supports, shoe raises, etc. Inspect the patient's footwear.
    ▶ Scars – back (laminectomy/microdiscectomy).
    ▶ Deformities (e.g. pes cavus).
    ▶ Muscle bulk – wasting.
    ▶ Tremors/fasciculations.
    ▶ Joints – swollen, erythematous.
    ▶ Posture – lumbar lordosis.
    ▶ Gait – footdrop (L5), broad-based (cerebellar).
    ▶ Romberg's test.

3 **Feel.**
    In the supine position:
    ▶ *Tone* – place hand on extended knee and rotate hip joint,
        briskly dorsiflex ankle and hold.
    ▶ *Sensation*:
        — groin/upper anterior thigh – L1
        — antero-lateral thigh – L2
        — medial thigh and knee – L3
        — medial calf – L4
        — lateral calf, foot dorsum, big toe – L5
        — sole of foot – S1
        — posterior calf and thigh – S2.
    ▶ Offer to test other sensory modalities (vibration, joint position
        sense, pain, temperature, etc.).

4 **Move.**
    ▶ *Power* (compare both sides):
        — hip flexors – try to push down straight leg flexed at hip (L2,
            L3)
        — hip extensors – ask patient to push leg into couch on to your
            hand (L5, S1)
        — knee flexors – try to extend flexed knee (L5, S1)

   — knee extensors – try to further flex semi-flexed knee (L3, L4)
   — foot dorsiflexors – try to push down upturned big toe (L5)
   — foot plantar flexors – ask the patient to push their foot down against your palm (S1, S2).

▮ *Coordination*:
   — heel to shin test.

▮ *Reflexes*:
   — knee – (L3/4, femoral nerve)
   — ankle – (S1/2, sciatic nerve)
   — clonus
   — Babinski reflex.

5 **Thank the patient and wash your hands.**

6 **Summarise and offer your differential diagnosis.**

LMN vs. UMN lesions

	LMN	UMN
Inspection	Wasting and atrophy	Normal muscle bulk
Fasciculations	Present	Absent
Tone	Decreases	Increases
Power	Decreases	Decreases
Reflexes	Absent/decreases	Increases

The circulatory system

'Please ask this patient some questions . . .': vascular system

Relevant questions to ask with regard to arterial disease include the following:

- patient's age and occupation
- intermittent claudication (site of pain – buttock, thigh, calf, precipitating and relieving factors)
- claudication distance and how it has varied with time (getting better, worse, or staying the same)
- back pain (*Note*: Be sure to distinguish vascular claudication from spinal stenosis/claudication)
- rest pain (including sleeping in a chair at night)
- ulceration, tissue loss
- gangrene
- history of cardiovascular disease (angina, myocardial infarcts, transient ischaemic attacks, strokes)
- cardiovascular risk factors – diabetes mellitus, smoking, hypertension, hypercholesterolaemia, previous history, family history
- previous vascular surgery
- functional status – impact on patient's life, walking aids, etc.
- fitness for surgery – anaesthetic history.

Relevant questions to ask with regard to venous disease include the following:

- patient's age and occupation
- discomfort, leg pain, heaviness
- itching around the ankles (eczema)
- skin pigmentation
- swelling/oedema
- bleeding varicose veins
- leg ulceration
- episodes of inflammation (pain/redness) over varicose veins (thrombophlebitis)
- history of DVTs, trauma to lower limbs, plaster casts (deep venous insufficiency)
- previous surgery for varicose veins, or where native veins have been utilised as grafts (e.g. CABG).

Approach to the ulcer

1 **Introduce yourself to the patient and wash your hands.**
Expose the whole limb.

Ask about pain. Noting the presence of pain also gives you a clue to the underlying aetiology (arterial vs. neuropathic).

2 **Inspect.**
   ▶ General – between the toes, tips of toes, pressure points, lift up the foot to inspect the heel, malleoli, under the fifth metatarsal head, ball of foot, amputations, and scars (legs and groin).
   ▶ Site, size (A × B cm), shape (regularly round or irregularly round) and number.

Then use the mnemonic **BEDD**:
   ▶ Base (healthy, slough, necrotic, avascular, malignant change, underlying structures such as tendon/muscle/fascia/bone/ligaments/joint visible).
   ▶ Edges (irregular/regular; sloping/punched out, etc.).
   ▶ Depth (in mm, or superficial/full thickness down to bone/tendon/fascia/muscle, etc.).
   ▶ Discharge (serous, sanguinous, serosanguinous, clear, purulent).
   ▶ Surrounding skin changes (chronic venous hypertension, other ulcers).
   ▶ Varicose veins.

3 **Palpation** (ask for gloves for this part of the examination!).
Temperature (assess with the back of the hand).
Tenderness.
Feel the base of the ulcer.

4 **Disease-specific tests.**
The commonest leg ulcers are venous, arterial, mixed and neuropathic. Test for each systematically. By now, however, you should have a pretty good idea which type of ulcer it is, so start with the most relevant tests first.

Arterial ulcers:
   ▶ Capillary refill around the ulcer.
   ▶ Pulses.

▶ Perform a complete arterial examination of the lower limbs (*see* 'Arterial examination of the lower limbs', page 72).

Neuropathic/diabetic ulcers:
  Test sensation.

Venous ulcers:
  Perform a full venous examination (*see* 'Venous examination of the lower limbs', page 76).

5 **Complete the examination.**
  ▶ Check the regional lymph nodes (infected and/or malignant ulcers). Are they tender?
  ▶ Auscultate for bruits.
  ▶ Test the urine for glucose.

6 **Thank the patient and wash your hands.**

7 **Summarise and offer your differential diagnosis.**

Differentiating the commonest types of leg ulcers

	Venous	Arterial	Neuropathic
Degree of pain	May be painful	Painful	Painless
Site	Gaiter area over medial malleolus	Tips of toes and pressure areas	Pressure areas (heel, malleoli, under metatarsal heads, tips of toes, between toes)
Size	Can be very large	Varying size (a few mm to several cm)	Several cm
Shape	Variable, usually irregular	Regular outline	Conform to shape of exposed pressure point
Base ulcer	Pink granulation tissue, or white fibrous tissue	No granulation tissue, bone may be exposed	Dry, often exposing bone or tendon
Edge ulcer	Sloping	Punched out, clean	Callous in edges, clean
Depth ulcer	Shallow	Often very deep. May penetrate down to deep fascia, tendon, bone, joint	Deep, penetrating
Surroundings	Varicose veins, varicose eczema, lipodermatosclerosis, oedema, haemosiderin deposition, atrophie blanche	Loss of peripheral pulses, pale/cold skin, hair loss, muscle wasting, venous guttering, amputations, gangrene, etc.	May be normal
Skin temperature	May be warmer	Cold	Normal
Pulses	Present	Absent pulses, prolonged capillary refill	Normal
Sensation	Present	Present	Absent

Arterial examination of the lower limbs

1 **Introduce yourself to the patient and wash your hands.**
Expose both limbs (with the socks removed), the abdomen and the chest.
   Check for tenderness.

2 **Inspect.**
   ▶ General – look for tar staining, carotid endarterectomy scars, median sternotomy scar (CABG), scars in the axilla (axillobifemoral bypass grafts), AAA, AAA scars, scars in the groin.
   ▶ Skin – look for nail changes for friability, skin colour, ulceration, gangrene, digital amputations/tissue loss, changes of coincidental venous disease, oedema (often due to dependency), hair loss, and venous guttering.
   ▶ SCARS from previous surgery (vein harvest, reconstruction procedures, grafts/flaps for soft tissue cover of ulcers and areas of tissue loss). Look for scars in the groin (exposure of common femoral artery).
   ▶ Muscles – wasted muscles (often due to disuse atrophy), loss of prominence of extensor tendons on the dorsum of the foot (oedema).
   ▶ Look in between the toes for changes.
   ▶ Ask the patient whether they have any pain, and then ask if you can lift the whole leg off the bed from the foot of the bed. Inspect the whole posterior aspect of the lower limb from the posterior thigh region right down to the heel, looking for ulcers, etc.
   ▶ Look for guttering of the veins.

3 **Palpate.**
   ▶ Temperature of the legs (start proximally, using the back of the hand, and compare one side with the other). Try to avoid feeling both sides simultaneously to compare the two sides, as the temperature of your hands may be different!
   ▶ Test for pitting oedema (usually secondary to dependency). Be gentle!
   ▶ Capillary refill (press the area for 5 seconds and the skin should flush within 2 seconds).

▶ Palpate for grafts in the medial thigh/groin.
▶ Palpate the pulses (note their presence or absence, the rate, rhythm, character and volume, as well as whether they are aneurysmal or not). Work from proximal to distal in a logical fashion. Feel one pulse at a time, with the tips of the fingers (the most sensitive part), and compare one side with the other. Try to avoid feeling both sides simultaneously to compare the two sides, as the examiners know that it is difficult to concentrate on two pulses simultaneously.
  — *Radial pulse* – rate and rhythm (if AF, consider embolic phenomenon).
  — *Abdominal aortic pulse* – palpate in the epigastrium for an AAA.
  — *Femoral pulse* – midway between the ASIS and the symphysis pubis at the mid-inguinal point. Palpate the radial pulse simultaneously to check for a radio-femoral delay.
  — *Popliteal pulse* – it is very important to get the patient to relax the hamstrings and calf muscles. Slightly flex the knee and wrap both hands around the knee, with the fingertips in the popliteal fossa and the thumbs of both hands on the tibial tuberosity. Compress the artery against the tibia posteriorly. Note that the popliteal pulse is often difficult to feel, unless aneurysmal, as the popliteal artery lies deep within the popliteal fossa. Feel for several beats and, if in doubt, compare the rate with your own pulse, as you can easily mistake the pulsations in your finger pulps for the popliteal pulse.
  — *Posterior tibial pulse* – behind the medial malleolus.
  — *Dorsalis pedis pulse* – felt between the head of the first and second metatarsals, or ask the patient to point their big toe to the ceiling and the pulsation may be felt just lateral to the tendon of the extensor hallucis longus. Note that the dorsalis pedis artery is congenitally absent in 10% of normal individuals, and this is usually bilateral.

4 **Auscultate.**
Bruits (AAA, renal, iliacs, femorals, adductor hiatus, popliteals). To examine for a bruit at the adductor hiatus, place the bell of your stethoscope at the surface anatomical landmark of the adductor

hiatus (also known as the subsartorial canal or Hunter's canal), which lies two-thirds of the way along a line drawn from the ASIS to the adductor tubercle.

5 **Buerger's test.**
Lift the patient's straight leg off the bed slowly (be gentle, and watch the patient's face at all times for signs of discomfort!). The angle of the leg from the bed when the leg turns white is Buerger's angle (if less than 20°, this indicates severe ischaemia). Help the patient to drop their leg over the side of the bed, and watch for reactive hyperaemia.

6 **ABPIs.**
Record the systolic pressure in both arms. Take the *higher* of the two readings. Then locate the dorsalis pedis and posterior tibial pulses with the handheld Doppler, and inflate the cuff until the Doppler sound disappears. Slowly deflate the cuff and record the pressure at which the sound reappears. Take the *higher* of the two readings (posterior tibial or dorsalis pedis). The ABPI is the ratio of the best foot systolic to brachial systolic pressure (normal, > 1.0; claudication, 0.4–0.7; critical ischaemia, 0.1–0.4).

7 **Complete the examination.**
  ▶ Test sensation (neurological status of the limb, to include nerves and muscles). Start distally. If they are insensate distally, work proximally until sensation returns. This is typical of the 'glove and stocking' distribution of sensory loss in the diabetic foot. Also offer to test the motor power, vibration sense, etc.
  ▶ Take a full history to determine the patient's functional status.
  ▶ Perform *Buerger's test*.
  ▶ Use hand-held Dopplers to determine presence of pulses and character of waveforms – i.e. normal triphasic, biphasic (moderate stenosis), monophasic (severe stenosis) or absent waveforms.
  ▶ Test ABPIs (at rest and during exercise) and examine the pulses after exercise.
  ▶ Offer an examination of the complete vascular tree, to include the heart, carotid arteries, blood pressure in both arms, etc.

▶ Test the urine for sugar/protein, and check the blood glucose level.
▶ Offer to perform fundoscopy to look for diabetic/hypertensive retinopathy.
▶ Offer to arrange a duplex USS.
▶ Offer to arrange an angiogram of the lower limbs.

8 Thank the patient and wash your hands.

9 Summarise and offer your differential diagnosis.

Venous examination of the lower limbs

We recommend that in addition to reading this section, you consult the following article:

▶ Bhasin N and Scott DJ. How should a candidate assess varicose veins in the MRCS examination? A vascular viewpoint. *Ann R Coll Surg Engl.* 2006; **88**: 309–12.

1 **Introduce yourself to the patient and wash your hands.**
   Stand the patient up and expose both limbs.
      Ask about pain.

2 **Inspect.**
   ▶ Ask the patient to stand with one leg in front of the other, and inspect from the front, sides and from behind.
   ▶ Look for varicose veins (abnormally prominent superficial, tortuous, dilated veins) and note their distribution (predominantly in the distribution of the long saphenous vein, the short saphenous vein, or both).
   ▶ Check for scars down the leg (avulsion sites).
   ▶ Check the groin for scars (previous high ligation and strip of long saphenous vein) and for a saphena varix.
   ▶ Check for haemangiomas and limb overgrowth (Klippel–Trenaunay syndrome, Parkes–Weber syndrome).

   Inspect the lower limbs for the following signs of *chronic venous hypertension*:
   ▶ ulceration
   ▶ haemosiderin staining/pigmentation
   ▶ venous eczema
   ▶ lipodermatosclerosis ('*inverted champagne bottle' leg*)
   ▶ oedema
   ▶ areas of healed ulceration (*atrophie blanche*), venous stars, and ankle flare (*corona phlebectatica*).

3 **Palpate.**
   ▶ Temperature – run the back of your hands up the legs, emptying the varicose veins to assess the compressibility and tortuosity, too.
      — Tenderness, induration, inflammation and thickening (thrombophlebitis).

— Hardening of the veins (thrombosis).
— Some varicosities can be better felt than seen.
— Pitting oedema (be gentle!).
— Defects in the fascia (site of incompetent perforators).
  Complete this in a stepwise, logical fashion, working from
  distal to proximal, in the course of the long and short
  saphenous veins, respectively).
— Saphena varix in groin.
— Cough test in groin (saphena varix). Feel for cough impulse/
  thrill.

4 **Percuss.**
Perform the *tap test* (also known as *Chevrier's percussion test*).
   Tap distally and feel proximally (orthograde transmission) to
assess venous continuity and venous patency, and to detect throm-
bosis/venous occlusion. Tap proximally and feel distally (retrograde
transmission) to detect venous valvular incompetence/reflux.

5 **Auscultate.**
Bruits may confirm arteriovenous fistulae.

6 **Special tests.**
   ▶ *The tourniquet test* (also known as the *Brodie–Trendelenburg test*
     if fingers or thumb are placed over the SFJ, instead of using a
     tourniquet). Elevate the limb to empty the veins. Then apply
     a tourniquet as high as possible on the upper thigh and stand
     the patient up. The veins will be controlled and will not fill
     if the incompetence is above the tourniquet site. If the veins
     refill, the incompetence is below the level of the tourniquet.
     This procedure should be repeated with the tourniquet
     positioned at a lower level on the thigh.
   ▶ The *hand-held Doppler* is used to assess incompetence at the
     sapheno-femoral and sapheno-popliteal junctions (ensure that
     the volume is turned up and that you use gel).

7 **Complete the examination.**
   ▶ Perform *Perthes' test* to assess the deep venous drainage.
   ▶ Perform a full arterial examination and ABPIs of the lower
     limb (before applying compression bandaging!).
   ▶ Take a full history to enquire about previous DVTs, trauma and

plaster casts, and to determine the effect of the venous disease on the patient's quality of life.

▶ Assess for causes of secondary varicose veins (perform an abdominal, pelvic examination, digital rectal examination, and examine the external genitalia).

▶ Offer to arrange a duplex Doppler examination of the lower limbs.

8 Thank the patient and wash your hands.

9 Summarise and offer your differential diagnosis.

Approach to the diabetic foot

1 **Introduce yourself to the patient and wash your hands.**
   Expose from the groin to the toes in the supine position, preserving the patient's dignity.
   Ask about pain (often absent in this scenario).

2 **Inspect.**
   ▶ General – cigarette tar stains, cardiovascular disease, insulin injection marks.
   ▶ Skin – colour, trophic changes, infection and ulcers, remembering to inspect the heel (site, size, edges, base, tender/pain, surrounding skin).

   Diabetic ulcers – on pressure points, smaller than venous ulcers, may be punched out, and may be infected, painless, with normal surrounding skin.
   ▶ Amputations.
   ▶ Ankle joint – Charcot joint.

3 **Palpation.**
   ▶ Temperature – run the back of your hand down the leg and foot and compare both sides.
   ▶ Capillary refill (small-vessel disease in diabetes mellitus).
   ▶ Sensation – test light touch over the dorsum of the foot, and if abnormal, move proximally to find the level where it becomes normal. Offer to test other sensory modalities (vibration sense, joint position sense, pain, temperature, etc.).

4 **Complete the examination.**
   ▶ Examine the patient for other signs of diabetes mellitus.
   ▶ Perform a complete cardiovascular examination, looking for concurrent cardiac and peripheral vascular disease (heart, carotid vessels, lower limbs). Beware of the fact that ABPIs are falsely elevated in diabetic patients due to calcification in the vessel wall.
   ▶ Perform fundoscopy to look for diabetic retinopathy.
   ▶ Check the blood sugar levels.
   ▶ Test the urine sugar levels.

5 Thank the patient and wash your hands.

6 Summarise and offer your differential diagnosis.

Examination of the AAA

1 Introduce yourself to the patient and wash your hands.
Ask the patient to lie flat on one pillow and expose the chest and abdomen.
  Ask about pain.

2 Inspect.
  ▶ Chest, neck and abdominal scars (e.g. midline sternotomy and carotid endarterectomy scars).
  ▶ Look for a pulsatile mass in the epigastrium.

3 Feel.
  ▶ To palpate for an AAA, perform *Fox's manoeuvre*, in two planes, with the hands flat on the epigastrium.
  ▶ Is the pulsatile mass expansile or transmitted? If there is an expansile rather than a transmitted pulsation, the fingers will be seen to be pushed apart in time with the pulsation of the aorta.
  ▶ Tenderness (AAAs are usually firm, non-tender, expansile and pulsatile swellings; tenderness implies imminent rupture, a leaking AAA, or an inflammatory aneurysm).
  ▶ Size of the AAA (diameter in cm) – by placing two hands on the abdominal wall, approaching from the sides. It is important to mention at this point that clinical examination is inaccurate for assessing the true size of an aneurysm, and that you would like to arrange an ultrasound scan, or CT, to determine the true aneurysm size.
  ▶ Can you get above it? If so, it is likely to be an infrarenal AAA.
  ▶ Can you get below it? If so, the AAA is unlikely to extend into the iliac vessels.

4 Auscultate.
Bruits – aortic, iliac, renal and femoral arteries.

5 The final steps.
  ▶ Check for coincidental femoral and popliteal aneurysms bilaterally.
  ▶ Check the distal pulses in the legs for thrombo-embolic complications.

6 **Complete the examination.**
Examine the rest of the cardiovascular system for concurrent cardiac and vascular disease (heart, carotid vessels, lower limbs).

7 **Thank the patient and wash your hands.**

8 **Summarise and offer your differential diagnosis.**

Arterial examination of the upper limbs

1 **Introduce yourself to the patient and wash your hands.**
  Obtain full exposure of the arms and chest – ask the patient to remove their shirt if necessary.
    Ask about pain.

2 **Inspect.**
  ▶ Tar staining.
  ▶ Nails – clubbing, brittle nails.
  ▶ Vasculitic changes.
  ▶ Pulp atrophy.
  ▶ Digital colour changes/cyanosis.
  ▶ Ulceration, gangrene or amputations.
  ▶ Muscle wasting.
  ▶ SCARS (arm, neck or midline sternotomy scars).
  ▶ Horner's syndrome.

3 **Feel.**
  ▶ Temperature.
  ▶ Capillary refill.
  ▶ Radial pulses (rate and rhythm) – radial, radio-radial delay, collapsing pulse (but check that there is no pain in the shoulder first, for the latter!).
  ▶ *Allen's test* (see below).

Allen's test is used to assess the relative contributions of the ulnar and radial arteries to the collateral blood supply of the hand.

To test the patency of the ulnar artery:
• Ask the patient to make a fist.
• Occlude both ulnar and radial pulses.
• Ask the patient to open their palm (which looks white).
• Release the ulnar artery. Does the palm become pink?

To test the patency of the radial artery:
• Ask the patient to make a fist.
• Occlude both ulnar and radial pulses.

> - Ask the patient to open their palm (which looks white).
> - Release the radial artery. Does the palm become pink?
>
> The sign is positive if the skin of the palm remains blanched for more than 5 seconds.

- ▶ Brachial pulse.
- ▶ Blood pressure in *both arms*.
- ▶ Palpate the axillary artery in the axilla (ask the patient to rest their hand on your forearm, as if palpating for axillary lymph nodes in a breast examination).
- ▶ Palpate the subclavian artery in the supraclavicular fossa (subclavian aneurysm, post-stenotic dilatation).
- ▶ Palpate the carotid artery (determine rate, rhythm, character and volume). Feel one artery at a time to prevent the patient from feeling dizzy.
- ▶ Palpate the superficial temporal artery (for signs of external carotid artery disease).
- ▶ Feel for a cervical rib.

4 **Auscultate.**
- ▶ Bruits in the supraclavicular fossa and infraclavicular space (subclavian).
- ▶ Carotid bruits (ask the patient to hold their breath; carotid bruits are best heard in expiration).

5 **Complete the examination.**
- ▶ Examine the rest of the cardiovascular system, including the lower limbs.
- ▶ Perform a neurological examination of the upper limb.
- ▶ Offer to perform special manoeuvres for thoracic outlet obstruction (*Adson's test*, *Wright's manoeuvre* and *Roos' test*).
- ▶ Perform fundoscopy to look for evidence of previous emboli.
- ▶ Request X-rays (CXR and C-spine to identify a cervical rib).

6 **Thank the patient and wash your hands.**

7 **Summarise and offer your differential diagnosis.**

Approach to the arteriovenous fistula

1 **Introduce yourself to the patient and wash your hands.**
Expose both arms.
   Ask about pain.

2 **Inspect.**
   ▶ Peripheral stigmata of end-stage renal disease.
   ▶ Any prominent swellings over the arm/forearm, arterialised veins, aneurysms.
   ▶ Distribution (radiocephalic, brachiocephalic, brachiobasilic).
   ▶ Non-dominant hand?
   ▶ Is the skin stretched over the surface?
   ▶ Overlying scars, needle marks overlying the swellings, e.g. haemodialysis access (if so, any swellings are likely to represent false aneurysms, or pseudoaneurysms).
   ▶ Visible pulsations.
   ▶ Ask the patient to raise their hand up in the air, and watch the veins empty.

3 **Feel.**
   ▶ Palpable thrill.
   ▶ Compressibility.
   ▶ Feel for loop grafts.
   ▶ Check the downstream pulses (with or without *Allen's test*).

4 **Percuss.**
Should be dull (fluid filled).

5 **Auscultate.**
Bruits (machinery murmur).

6 **The final steps.**
   ▶ Check for complications in the hand ('steal phenomenon', swelling secondary to venous hypertension).
   ▶ Perform *Allen's test*

7 **Complete the examination.**
   ▶ Check the neck and chest for Tesio lines (for haemodialysis/vascular access), or scars from previous Tesio lines.

> ▶ Check the abdomen for Tenckhoff catheters for peritoneal dialysis (or evident scars from previous catheter sites).
> ▶ Check the abdomen for masses (renal transplant, renal masses such as polycystic kidneys) and scars (nephrectomy, transplant scars).

8 Thank the patient and wash your hands.

9 Summarise and offer your differential diagnosis.

Approach to the amputation

When examining an amputee, it is helpful to remember the properties of an ideal amputation stump:

▶ The stump heals by primary wound intention.
▶ There is no redundant tissue.
▶ The stump is cylindrical.
▶ There is no pressure on the suture line.
▶ The stump is painless.
▶ There is full extension and flexion in adjacent joints.

1 **Introduce yourself to the patient and wash your hands.**
   Expose both legs and the abdomen in the supine position or with the patient seated in a chair (as presented), preserving the patient's dignity.
   Ask about pain (don't forget *phantom limb pain*!).

2 **Look.**
   ▶ Level of amputation: below knee (14 cm below knee), above knee (12 cm above knee), hindquarter, Gritti–Stokes and through knee, Syme's, Chopart's (at mid-tarsal joint), Lisfranc's (at tarso-metatarsal joint), transmetatarsal, Ray, digital, etc. (*see* Figure 2).
   ▶ Stump type – cylindrical shape (for below knee – long posterior flap of Burgess, or skew flap of Kingsley Robinson).
   ▶ Stump viability – healing, infection, necrosis, ulceration.
   ▶ Prostheses.
   ▶ Scars from previous surgery.

3 **Feel.**
   ▶ Capillary refill (< 2 seconds).
   ▶ Assess whether the soft tissues move freely over bone.
   ▶ Feel for bony spurs and osteophytes in the underlying bone.
   ▶ Palpate the pulses (for further ischaemia, which may require revision surgery).

4 **Move (active then passive).**
   ▶ Ask the patient to actively flex and extend the hip joint and/or knee joint if it is a below-knee amputation, to check for fixed flexion deformities.

▶ Perform passive flexion and extension (if the patient cannot actively bend).

▶ Ask the patient to fit any prostheses and walk.

5. **Complete the examination.**

▶ Examine the other limb for signs of peripheral vascular disease.

▶ Perform a full cardiovascular and respiratory examination to assess risks for surgery.

6 **Thank the patient and wash your hands.**

7 **Summarise and offer your differential diagnosis.**

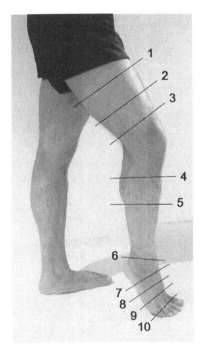

Figure 2: Amputation levels. 1. Short above knee, 2. Medium above knee, 3. Long above knee, 4. Short below knee, 5. Standard below knee, 6. Syme's, 7. Chopart, 8. Lisfranc, 9. Transmetatarsal, 10. Ray, Digital

The abdomen, trunk and groin

The abdominal examination

1 **Introduce yourself to the patient and wash your hands.**

Lie the patient flat on the bed with one pillow.

Obtain adequate exposure from nipples to knees, keeping the genital area covered unless you are asked to examine that area.

Ask about pain.

2 **Inspect (general and specific).**

Inspection should begin from the foot of the bed, looking 'from out to in' – that is, looking around the bed for clues first, and then looking at the patient (for signs, such as jaundice and cachexia). Still from the foot of the bed, inspect the abdomen for the following:

▶ Is the abdomen moving freely with respiration?

▶ Ask the patient to push their abdomen out and suck it back in. Look at the patient's face for signs of discomfort.

▶ Distension (central or in flanks?).

▶ Ask the patient to cough.

▶ Ask the patient to lift their head off the bed, or to lift both legs together off the bed. Look at the patient's face for signs of pain, and look for abdominal wall hernias.

Approach the patient from their right side for closer inspection.

▶ Start with the hands – look for clubbing, leukonychia, paronychia, palmar erythema, pallor in the palmar creases, Dupuytren's contracture, pulse.

▶ Arms – look for liver flap, scratch marks related to pruritus.

▶ Eyes – look for icterus and pallor (*Note*: pull both eyelids down together).

▶ Mouth – look for jaundice (palate and lower surface of tongue), ulcers, state of dentition, tongue changes. Ask the patient to lift their tongue up, and look for telangiectasia.

▶ Neck – check for supraclavicular lymph nodes (Virchow's node/Troisier's sign).

▶ Chest – look for spider naevi, gynaecomastia, scratch marks.

Inspect the abdomen from close up.

▶ Central – umbilical shape (paraumbilical hernias are easily missed!), dilated veins.

▶ The flanks – distension/fullness.

- Check carefully for scars and fistulae, quadrant by quadrant. Multiple scars of different ages often suggest Crohn's disease.
- Ask the patient to roll to each side so that you can visualise the loins/renal angles for any scars or masses.
- Get down level with the abdomen to look for masses, visible peristalsis and AAA pulsations (ask the patient to hold their breath while you look for the latter).

3 **Palpation.**

Ask the patient to point with one finger to the area that is most painful. Ensure that you have clean, warm hands and nails that are cut short.

- Perform superficial palpation first – four quadrants and central area to check for tenderness and obvious masses (*you must keep your eyes fixed on the patient's face at all times to detect signs of tenderness*).
- Deep palpation – nine areas for masses.
- Feel for a liver edge – start in the RIF, and as the patient breathes in deeply move up towards the costal margin.
- Feel for the spleen – start in the RIF moving up towards the left costal margin, as the patient breathes in. To detect a mildly enlarged spleen, roll the patient over to their right-hand side.
- Ballott the kidneys.
- To detect an AAA, feel for an expansile, pulsatile mass in the epigastrium, in two planes, with the hands flat on the abdomen (*Fox's manoeuvre*). If there is an expansile rather than a transmitted pulsation, the fingers will be seen to be pushed apart in time with the pulsation of the aorta.

4 **Percussion.**

- Elicit the presence or absence of peritoneal irritation.
- Assess the size of the liver from the fifth intercostal space, mid-clavicular line downwards.
- Assess the size of the spleen from the RIF.
- Percuss the bladder in the suprapubic area.
- Percuss for free fluid/ascites (with or without fluid thrill, shifting dullness).

5 **Auscultate.**

- Bowel sounds.

- Renal bruits.
- Venous hums.
- Friction rubs.
- Femoral artery bruits.

6 **Groin and ankles.**
- Place one hand on each superficial ring and ask the patient to cough (hernia).
- Place one hand on each deep ring and ask the patient to cough (hernia).
- Palpate for groin lymph nodes.
- Check for ankle oedema.

7 **Complete the examination.**
- Offer to examine the external genitalia.
- Offer to perform a digital rectal examination.
- Check the urine and dipstick test.
- Check the stool chart (if appropriate).
- Check the observation and fluid balance charts.

8 **Thank the patient and wash your hands.**

9 **Summarise and offer your differential diagnosis.**
If you identify any abdominal scar during the exam, comment on the:
- age (old or recent)
- healing tendency (well healed or poorly healed)
- complications of the scar itself (infected, hypertrophic, atrophic or keloid)
- associated complications of the wound (incisional hernia, false aneurysm, etc.)
- presence or absence of drain site scars and stoma scars in the surroundings.

Approach to the abdominal lump

1 **Introduce yourself to the patient and wash your hands.**
Lie the patient flat on the bed with one pillow.
Ask about pain.

2 Inspection/palpation/percussion/auscultation.
   ▶ Site.
   ▶ Scars overlying it (e.g. renal transplant).
   ▶ Size.
   ▶ Shape.
   ▶ Surface – regular or irregular.
   ▶ Edge – regular or irregular.
   ▶ Tenderness.
   ▶ Temperature.
   ▶ Consistency.
   ▶ Can you get above and below it?
   ▶ Pinch the skin over it.
   ▶ Ask the patient to lift their head off the bed, or to lift both feet up in the air to tense the rectus sheath. Determine the relationship of the lump to the muscle and the mobility/fixity (*Carnett's test*) (*see* 'Approach to any lump (or cutaneous lesion)', page 12).
   ▶ Cough impulse.
   ▶ Reducibility/compressibility.
   ▶ Fluctuance.
   ▶ Pulsatility and expansility.
   ▶ Does it move with respiration?
   ▶ Can it be ballotted?
   ▶ Percuss the lump.
   ▶ Auscultate over the lump.
   ▶ Palpate for regional lymph nodes (inguinal and axillary, especially if the case is splenomegaly), and check the neurovascular status.

Note: In the case of hepatomegaly:
   ▶ Determine how far the liver extends beneath the costal margin (cm/finger breadths).
   ▶ Percuss the upper border of the liver to demonstrate that it has not been pushed down by hyperexpanded lungs.

> ▶ Assess liver consistency (soft, firm, hard, craggy).
> ▶ Comment on the liver edge (smooth or nodular).
> ▶ Assess liver tenderness.
> ▶ Assess liver pulsatility.
> ▶ Don't forget the Reidel's lobe!

3 **Thank the patient and wash your hands.**

4 **Summarise and offer your differential diagnosis.**

Common causes of hepatomegaly and splenomegaly
Isolated hepatomegaly

Physiological causes:
- Riedel's lobe
- hyperexpanded chest (liver ptosis).

Alcoholic liver disease:
- fatty liver
- macronodular cirrhosis.

Neoplastic disease:
- benign – polycystic kidney disease, hepatomas
- primary – hepatocellular carcinoma, angiosarcoma, cholangiocarcinoma
- secondary – metastatic deposits, lymphoma, myeloproliferative disorders.

Infections:
- viral – viral hepatitis, EBV, CMV, HIV
- bacterial – TB, liver abscess
- protozoal – malaria, hydatid, amoebiasis, schistosomiasis.

Congestive cardiac failure.

Metabolic diseases and infiltrative diseases:
- Wilson's disease, haemochromatosis, Gaucher's disease
- amyloidosis, sarcoidosis.

Isolated splenomegaly

Haematological disease:
- benign – haemolytic anaemias, pernicious anaemia, idiopathic thrombocytopaenic purpura, sickle-cell disease (early stages)
- malignant – myeloproliferative and lymphoproliferative disorders.

Portal hypertension – pre-sinusoidal, sinusoidal, post-sinusoidal causes.

Infections:
- viral – EBV, CMV, HIV

- bacterial – typhoid, typhus, TB, sepsis, bacterial endocarditis
- protozoal – malaria, schistosomiasis, kala-azar.

Space-occupying lesions:
- solitary cysts, polycystic disease.

Cellular infiltration and systemic diseases:
- amyloidosis, rheumatoid arthritis (Felty's syndrome), Gaucher's disease, SLE, sarcoidosis.

Hepatosplenomegaly

- Portal hypertension.
- Myeloproliferative disorders.
- Lymphoproliferative disorders.

Distinguishing a spleen from a kidney clinically

	Spleen	Left kidney
Descent on inspiration	Towards right iliac fossa	Vertically
Ballottable (bimanually palpable)?	No	Yes
Notch present	Yes	No
Can you get above it?	No	Sometimes
Percussion note	Dull	Usually resonant (overlying bowel)
Friction rub	Occasionally	No

Stigmata of chronic liver disease

Hands:

▶ leukonychia, clubbing, palmar erythema, Dupuytren's contracture, bruising, asterixis (flapping tremor), pruritus/scratch marks.

Face:

▶ jaundice, scratch marks, spider naevi, foetor hepaticus.

Chest:

▶ gynaecomastia, loss of body hair, spider naevi, bruising, pectoral muscle wasting.

Abdomen:

▶ signs of portal hypertension (hepatosplenomegaly, ascites, caput medusae), testicular atrophy.

Legs:

▶ oedema, muscle wasting, bruising.

Approach to the stoma

1 **Introduce yourself to the patient and wash your hands.**
Lie the patient flat on the bed with one pillow, obtaining adequate exposure from nipples to knees.
  Ask about pain.

2 **Inspect the stoma.**
  ▶ In which quadrant is it sited?
  ▶ Look for scars throughout the abdomen (previous surgery and stomas).
  ▶ Check the contents of the bag (liquid faeces, formed faeces, urine).
  ▶ Is the stoma flush or spout with the skin (ileostomy vs. colostomy)?
  ▶ Is the stoma single- or double-lumen (end vs. loop stoma)?
  ▶ If it is a loop stoma, look for the presence of a bridge (a newly formed stoma).
  ▶ If the patient has a loop stoma, identify the afferent and efferent limbs of the stoma. The *afferent limb*, or functional end, produces the stool output and is usually larger and more caudally placed to prevent spill-over into the efferent limb. The *efferent* limb allows passage of flatus and mucous discharge from the distal, 'defunctioned' portion of the bowel, and is usually smaller and more cephalic.

  Look for complications:
  ▶ Does the stoma look healthy? (Avoid using the phrase 'The stoma looks nice', as it isn't nice for the patient! It would be better to say 'The stoma looks healthy and is well fashioned').
  ▶ Is it well sited (i.e. placed away from scars, bony prominences and skin folds)?
  ▶ Ask the patient to cough and lift their head off the bed so that you can check for the presence of a parastomal hernia.
  ▶ Look for prolapse, retraction, mucocutaneous separation, ischaemia/necrosis, ulceration, stenosis, oedema, parastomal hernia and high output.
  ▶ Look at the surrounding skin for excoriation and erythema which may be due to a poorly fitting bag.

3 Palpation.
   ▶ Offer to insert a finger into the stoma to check stoma patency and stenosis. First check that the patient can reapply the stoma bag.
   ▶ Offer to shine a light down into the stoma to check that the mucosa is healthy.

4 Complete the examination.
   ▶ Inspect the perineum for scars and the presence of an anal opening.
   ▶ Offer to perform a complete abdominal examination.
   ▶ Assess the position of the stoma with the patient sitting, lying and standing.

5 Thank the patient and wash your hands.

6 Summarise and offer your differential diagnosis.

7 Try to offer an explanation for the need for the stoma in the first place.

Examination of the groin

1 **Introduce yourself to the patient and wash your hands.**
Ideally stand the patient up and obtain full exposure of the groin, genitalia and abdomen. However, be prepared to be flexible. For example, if you are asked to examine the groin, and the patient is an elderly man sitting in a wheelchair, the examiners will not be impressed if you try to get him to stand up!
Ask about pain and tell the patient that you will be gentle.

Note: Each time that you ask the patient to cough, this should have a specific purpose. The examiners will be watching carefully how many times you make the patient cough and at which stage.

2 **Inspect.**
  ▶ Look for any lumps in the groin and define their characteristics.
  ▶ Look carefully for scars, especially overlying any lumps.
  ▶ Ask the patient to look away and cough. Look at the superficial ring of the affected side for a cough impulse (*cough 1*). Then ask the patient to cough again and look at the contralateral/normal side (*cough 2*).

3 **Palpate.**
  ▶ Can you get above the lump? If you cannot, it is indeed likely to be a groin swelling and you should proceed as described below. If you can get above the lump, it is likely to be a scrotal lump (*see* 'Examination of the scrotum', page 104).

4 **The 'Insider Medical' hernia protocol.**
  Step 1: Where is the lump? (Define the anatomy and its relations)
  ▶ Stand to the side of the patient with one hand on their back and the other hand on the lump itself.
  ▶ Identify key landmarks (ASIS, pubic tubercle, the interposed inguinal ligament, femoral artery pulsation, etc.).
  ▶ Define the relationship of the lump to the pubic tubercle (femoral vs. inguinal hernia) and the inguinal ligament.

  Step 2: What is it like? (Define the characteristics of the lump)
  Define the characteristics of the lump in the groin, as you would

for any other lump anywhere else (*see* 'Approach to any lump (or cutaneous lesion)', page 12).

Step 3: Confirm that it is a hernia (Expansile cough impulse, reducibility, bowel sounds)
▶ With your hand on the lump, ask the patient to look away and cough (*cough 3*). Is there an expansile cough impulse?
▶ Assess for reducibility. Ask the patient whether the lump 'ever goes back inside.' If so, ask the patient to push it back in for you: '*Can you push it back in for me and make the lump disappear?*'

Watch how the patient reduces it (straight back, implying a direct inguinal hernia, or following an oblique course backwards and laterally, implying an indirect inguinal hernia).
  If the lump is difficult to reduce at any stage, lie the patient down.
▶ Place one finger on the pubic tubercle and ask the patient to cough again (*cough 4*). Note the relationship of the lump to the pubic tubercle as it protrudes:
    — above and medial to the pubic tubercle suggests inguinal hernia
    — below and lateral to the pubic tubercle suggests femoral hernia.

Step 4: Is the inguinal hernia direct or indirect?
Perform the *deep ring occlusion test*. Place one hand on the deep inguinal ring, situated just above a point halfway between the pubic tubercle and the ASIS, and then ask the patient to look away and cough (*cough 5*). If the lump is controlled at the level of the deep ring, the inguinal hernia is indirect.

Step 5: Check that the bowel is alive!
Auscultate for bowel sounds.

5 **The final steps.**
▶ Examine the contralateral groin.
▶ Examine the scrotum on both sides. (There may be a coincidental hydrocele or varicocele, etc. The likelihood of dual pathologies featuring in the MRCS exam is far higher than in everyday clinical practice!)

▶ Offer to stand the patient up if you have not already done so (to avoid missing a varicocele).

6 Complete the examination.
▶ Examine the regional lymph nodes.
▶ Offer to take a full history.
▶ Offer to examine the abdomen.
▶ Offer to perform a digital rectal examination.
▶ Offer to assess the cardiovascular and respiratory systems with the patient's fitness for surgery in mind.

7 Thank the patient and wash your hands.

8 Summarise and offer your differential diagnosis. For example:

'This is a well-looking, middle-aged man, who has a 2 × 2 cm non-tender, fully reducible lump in the left groin that lies above and medial to the pubic tubercle. It has an expansile cough impulse and is controlled by pressure over the deep/internal inguinal ring. These findings support a diagnosis of a left-sided indirect inguinal hernia. The contralateral side and genitalia are normal. To complete my examination I would like to take a full history, examine the abdomen, and assess this patient's fitness for surgery by performing a full cardio-respiratory history and examination.'

When formulating a differential diagnosis in the exam, try to think anatomically. What structures are present in the vicinity of the problem? It may be helpful to sieve through the layers from the skin. The differential diagnosis of a groin lump may therefore include:
▶ skin – *sebaceous cyst*
▶ subcutaneous tissues – *lipoma, fibroma*
▶ lymphatics – *inguinal lymphadenopathy*
▶ bowel – *inguinal, femoral hernia*
▶ vein – *saphena varix*
▶ artery – *femoral artery aneurysm*
▶ nerve – *neuroma, neurofibroma*
▶ spermatic cord – *lipoma of the cord, encysted hydrocele of cord*
▶ testis/scrotum – *ectopic testis*
▶ muscle – *benign/malignant tumour (sarcoma)*
▶ psoas sheath – *psoas abscess, psoas bursa.*

Examination of the scrotum

1 **Introduce yourself to the patient and wash your hands.**

Ideally stand the patient up and obtain full exposure of the groin, genitalia and abdomen. However, be prepared to be flexible. For example, if you are asked to examine the groin, and the patient is an elderly man sitting in a wheelchair, the examiners will not be impressed if you try to get him to stand up!

Ask about pain, and explain to the patient that you will be gentle.

2 **Inspect.**
  ▶ Ask the patient to look away and cough.
  ▶ Inspect for groin and scrotal scars (including the posterior aspect of the scrotum).

3 **Palpate.**
  ▶ Can you get above the lump? If you can, the lump is a true scrotal lump and you should proceed as described below. If you cannot, the lump is in fact arising from the groin, e.g. an inguino-scrotal hernia (*see* 'Examination of the groin', page 101).
  ▶ Is the testis separable from the lump?
  ▶ Define the characteristics of the lump, as you would for any other lump.
  ▶ Does the lump transilluminate?
  ▶ Does the scrotal skin move easily over the lump?
  ▶ Ask the patient to cough. Is there a cough impulse?
  ▶ Examine the abdomen for para-aortic nodes.
  ▶ Don't forget to examine *both* testes!
  ▶ Offer to stand the patient up if you have not done so already (to avoid missing a varicocele.)

4 **Complete the examination.**
  ▶ Offer to take a full history.
  ▶ Offer to examine the abdomen.
  ▶ Offer to perform a digital rectal examination.

5 **Thank the patient and wash your hands.**

6 **Summarise and offer your differential diagnosis.**

SECTION B

Communication skills for the MRCS clinical exam

Top tips for communication skills

Communication skills are an inherent skill required by doctors to distribute important information to patients and their families, and to fellow colleagues. This process encompasses both verbal and non-verbal communication techniques to convey and receive information in a structured and well thought out manner.

Environment

Select a tranquil environment, in which interruptions can be avoided. Ensure that your pager or bleep is either turned off or left outside the consultation room. Consider rearranging the furniture (including chairs) to ensure that you are sitting at the level of the patient and not across a desk from them. Allow the patient to have a sense of equality during the communication and not to feel overawed or intimidated by their surroundings.

Introduction

Greet the patient or relative by telling them your name and position. Establish the name of the person to whom you are talking – don't make any assumptions. Ensure that you have consent from the patient if you are communicating with a member of their extended family. Ask the patient or relative whether they wish to be alone or accompanied by a friend, family member or nurse.

Consultation

Establish what the patient and/or family member understands about the patient's current medical condition. Employ verbal and non-verbal communication techniques to establish clear communication skills and overall patient satisfaction.

Non-verbal communication techniques

Your body language is an important aid to the free flow of communication. It is best to sit in a neutral position (i.e. without your arms or legs crossed or standing over the patient or relative). Establish good eye contact. Demonstrate that you are 'actively' listening – for example, by repeating the salient points of what has been communicated and clarifying certain issues.

Make use of silences and pauses to enable the patient or relative to express their true concerns. Positive movements such as nodding and smiling (if appropriate) will allow the communicator to feel comfortable in this environment.

Verbal communication techniques

Start with open-ended questions, and then proceed with direct and closed questions. For clear and effective communication, use simple language and avoid using medical jargon or abbreviations in order to minimise confusion and misunderstandings. Address the *ideas, concerns and expectations (ICE)* of the patient or relative. You will need to consider the patient's psychological and social concerns. They may have already formed an opinion and have an underlying agenda which you must uncover and address. An important tip is to re-check the understanding of the patient or relative as you go along.

If the patient or relative is tearful, show empathy by providing tissues. If there has been a misunderstanding or a mistake, you may apologise. If they are angry or aggressive, attempt to understand the reasons for this in order to ameliorate the stressful situation.

Illustrations (i.e. pictures and diagrams) and patient information leaflets can be used as helpful aids to demonstrate the salient features of your discussion.

It is important to establish a multi-disciplinary approach by encompassing other specialties (i.e. medical and surgical colleagues, physiotherapists, occupational therapists, social workers and nurse specialists) during your consultation.

Conclusion

Summarise what has been communicated, ensure that the patient or relative has a clear understanding, and provide a future management plan. Establish whether the patient or relative has any further concerns or questions. Finally, repeat your name and position along with your contact details to enable the patient or relative to contact you in the future. If appropriate, make a further appointment.

The exam format
Information giving

In this part of the examination, you will be given a total of 5 minutes to spend reading through a clinical scenario, and then a total of 10 minutes to communicate with a patient and/or their relative. The objective of this station is to deliver the required information effectively. The examiners will be present throughout the entire interview. They will not interrupt your communication, but will be present to mark your performance.

Common scenarios include *breaking bad news*, explaining an operation (*consent*) and communicating with angry relatives (*complaints*). During your 5 minutes of preparation time, try to anticipate how the patient will be feeling, what their concerns may be, what they will want to know and what questions they may have.

Information gathering

In this part of the examination, you will be required to gather information from a patient and/or their relative. History taking is essential to guide future investigation, obtain a diagnosis and implement treatment. The exact scenario will be provided prior to consultation with the patient and/or relative.

The overall objectives of this station will be to take a focused surgical history, establish a differential diagnosis, explain what clinical signs would be present on the clinical examination, list the essential investigations and finally provide a treatment plan (including conservative, medical or surgical options).

You will be given 5 minutes to review the case and a further 10 minutes to obtain the required information. At the end of the 10 minutes, a bell will sound. The actor/actress will then leave the room and you will be required to present the case to your two consultant examiners and answer their questions relating to the differential diagnosis, clinical signs you would look for on examination, investigations and treatment options. During the latter part of the examination, you are specifically being assessed on the delivery of your presentation and your communication with professional colleagues.

Make the best possible use of the 5 minutes of preparation time by trying to think about what questions you are going to ask the patient. Try to predict how the patient may be feeling and what concerns they may have. Think about how you will deal with the patient who is very anxious, aggressive, timid, distressed, withdrawn or embarrassed, or who will not stop talking!

Although you are provided with paper in the examination, try to avoid writing anything down, otherwise eye contact and non-verbal cues will be compromised. If this is something you are not used to, then we recommend that you practise history taking and presenting to your consultant without the aid of pen and paper prior to the exam. When you present to the examiners, speak slowly and make good eye contact.

History taking
▶ Personal details
▶ Presenting complaint
▶ History of presenting complaint
   — System-specific questions
   — Risk factors for the presenting complaint
   — Investigations and treatment to date
▶ Past medical, surgical and anaesthetic history
▶ Medication and known allergies
▶ Family history
▶ Social history
▶ Review of systems

Marking scheme
The examiner will score each consultation on a scale of 1 (lowest possible score) to 4 (highest possible score).

Insider's communication framework

1 Preparation
2 Introduction
3 Consultation
4 Consolidation
5 Conclusion

Clinical scenarios: information giving

Case 1: Breaking bad news

As the surgical trainee in general surgery, you are required to speak to Mrs Brown and her husband about her recent investigation in the one-stop breast clinic. She has undergone triple assessment for a breast lump. She must be informed that she been diagnosed with carcinoma of the breast.

Preparation

Ensure that you have read the patient's medical notes and confirm the diagnosis. If possible have the breast care nurse available. You are required to inform Mrs Brown about her diagnosis and formulate a management plan.

Introduction

Introduce yourself to the patient and her husband.

Consultation

First, establish what Mrs Brown understands about her condition. She explains that she found a breast lump 2 weeks ago and that she has undergone a series of investigations to find out what it is. She is afraid that it may be cancer, as her mother had breast cancer. Once this background information has been obtained, you inform her that she does indeed have breast cancer. Do not try to avoid using the word 'cancer.' It is essential to show compassion. You will need to explain that further staging will be performed, and that she will need surgery and further treatment. Be patient and give the patient an opportunity to absorb this information. A standard approach and useful mnemonic for breaking bad news is **SPIKES** (Buckman R *et al.* SPIKES – a six step protocol for delivering bad news. *The Oncologist* 2000; **5**: 302– 11)

Set Stage and Setting
Patient Perception
Invitation
Knowledge
Explore Emotions and Empathise
Strategy and Summary

Consolidation

Reiterate the key points of this consultation. Allow time for any questions to be addressed by the patient and her husband.

Conclusion

Provide Mrs Brown with a clear management plan and follow-up. Establish when further treatment will commence. Provide information leaflets and support group contact details. Provide your own contact numbers to ensure that the patient can communicate with you about any concerns or questions that they may have. In addition, ensure that the breast cancer nurse is fully informed.

Case 2: Breaking bad news

As the surgical trainee on call, you are required to speak to the daughter of Mrs Smith, who was admitted for a fracture of the neck of femur. She underwent a dynamic hip screw without complication. However, she has now been diagnosed with a deep vein thrombosis (DVT).

Preparation

Ensure that you have read the patient's medical notes. You are required to address why Mrs Smith's operation was necessary, her post-operative complications and further treatment required.

Introduction

A full introduction is needed, as you have not met Mrs Smith's daughter.

Consultation

First, establish what the daughter already knows about her mother's condition. Once this background information has been obtained, provide information about the underlying hip fracture, the operation and post-operative complications. Explain what a deep venous thrombosis is, and its associated risk factors according to Virchow's triad – blood flow (stasis), vessel wall (compression, trauma) and blood constituents (hyperviscosity, hypercoagulability). Then explain the recommended course of treatment (including anticoagulation) for Mrs Smith. In addition, you need to explain the severity of her condition and the potential risk of morbidity and mortality. A standard approach is listed below:

Set Stage and Setting
Patient Perception
Invitation
Knowledge
Explore Emotions and Empathise
Strategy and Summary

Consolidation

Reiterate the key points of this consultation. Allow time for the daughter to raise any concerns or questions.

Conclusion

Provide the daughter with a clear management plan. Establish when further information will be available. Provide contact numbers to ensure that the family can contact the nursing and medical teams to arrange further consultations.

Case 3: Breaking bad news

As the surgical trainee, you are required to speak to Mr Harris, who was admitted following a serious motorcycle accident. Mr Harris must be informed that, based on the severity of his injuries, he requires a lower limb amputation.

Preparation

Ensure that you have read Mr Harris's medical notes. You are required to explain the necessity for the amputation, the potential complications, and further treatment.

Introduction

A full introduction is required.

Consultation

First, establish what Mr Harris understands about his condition. Once this information has been obtained, you can provide him with the management plan. Explain that other options have been explored (i.e. reconstruction), but based on the severity of his injuries an amputation is the only option available. Allow the patient ample time to digest this distressing news. Explain the benefits and potential complications of the operation. Following his operation, Mr Harris will undergo rehabilitation. A standard approach is listed below:

Set Stage and Setting
Patient Perception
Invitation
Knowledge
Explore Emotions and Empathise
Strategy and Summary

Consolidation

Reiterate the key points of this consultation. Allow time for concerns or questions that Mr Harris may have.

Conclusion

Provide Mr Harris with a clear management plan. Establish when further information will be available, and provide him with your contact details.

Case 4: Consent

As the surgical trainee on call, you are required to speak to Mr Tracey. It has been recommended that he should have an anterior resection for rectal cancer under general anaesthetic.

Preparation

Ensure that you have read the patient's medical notes and confirmed the diagnosis. You will be expected to discuss the aims, benefits, potential complications of and alternatives to a resection. Also provide information about the potential risks of surgery in general, specific to the operation, and of the anaesthetic. To obtain informed consent you must provide the patient with sufficient information so that he can weigh up the available options and make an informed decision.

Introduction

A full introduction is required.

Consultation

First, establish what the patient understands about his condition and the operation. Explain the anterior resection (i.e. a surgical procedure conducted under general anaesthetic that removes a portion of large bowel, and the two ends of bowel are then rejoined, the aim of this operation being to remove a portion of diseased bowel). Explain the potential complications (i.e. infection, bleeding, recurrence, resection failure, the need for further surgery, damage to surrounding structures, stoma formation, complications of general anaesthetics, risk to life, etc.). A standard approach and useful mnemonic for consenting any patient for any operation is **CONSENTS**:

Condition and natural history
Options and alternatives (i.e conservative, medical or surgical)
Name of procedure; Not to treat
Side-effects/complications (i.e. anaesthetic, infection, bleeding, recurrence, stoma formation, etc.)
Extra procedures (i.e. drain/nasogastric tube/catheter/PCA insertion, stoma formation, blood transfusion)
Named person operating
Trial and Training (i.e. research and students)
Second opinion

Consolidation

Reiterate the key points of this consultation. Allow time to address any concerns or questions that Mr Tracey may have. Finally, ask him to sign the consent form.

Conclusion

Provide Mr Tracey with a copy of his consent form, information leaflets and support group contact details. You should also provide him with your own contact information.

Case 5: Consent

As the surgical trainee on call, you are required to speak to Mrs Rogers. She is scheduled for a colonoscopy under sedation.

Preparation

Ensure that you have read the patient's medical notes. You will be expected to discuss the aims, benefits, potential complications of and alternatives to this procedure. To obtain informed consent you must provide the patient with sufficient information so that they can weigh up the available options and make an informed decision.

Introduction

A full introduction is required. Confirm that Mrs Rogers has taken the prescribed bowel preparation and that she is 'nil by mouth.'

Consultation

First, establish what Mrs Rogers understands about her condition and the procedure. Explain what a colonoscopy is (i.e. a procedure to visualise the large bowel, obtain a diagnosis and provide treatment). Explain the potential complications (i.e. infection, bleeding, bowel perforation, failure to perform the procedure or obtain a histological diagnosis, etc.). A standard approach is listed below:

Condition and natural history
Options and alternatives (i.e. radiological: CT scan or barium enema)
Name of procedure; Not to treat
Side-effects
Extra procedures (i.e. biopsy)
Named person operating
Trial and Training (i.e. research and students)
Second opinion

Consolidation

Reiterate the key points of this consultation. Allow time to address any concerns or questions that Mrs Rogers may have. Finally, ask her to sign the consent form.

Conclusion

Provide Mrs Rogers with a copy of her consent form, information leaflets and support group contact details. You should also provide her with your own contact information.

Case 6: Consent

As the surgical trainee on call, you are required to speak to Mrs Lee. She was admitted with a sudden-onset headache, photophobia and neck stiffness. A lumbar puncture is required.

Preparation

Ensure that you have read the patient's medical notes. You will be expected to discuss the aims, benefits, potential complications of and alternatives to this procedure. To obtain informed consent, you must provide the patient with sufficient information so that they can weigh up the available options and make an informed decision.

Introduction

A full introduction is required.

Consultation

First, establish what Mrs Lee understands about her condition and the procedure. Explain the lumbar puncture and its indications:

▶ *diagnostic* – to obtain a sample of CSF for assessment of infection (meningitis), blood (subarachnoid haemorrhage), malignant cells and abnormal proteins (myeloma)

▶ *therapeutic* – to administer intrathecal drugs (chemotherapy, antibiotics).

Explain the contraindications to a lumbar puncture (raised intracranial pressure – if you suspect this, perform a CT scan of the head before proceeding), localised infection, coagulopathy or a suspected spinal cord or posterior fossa mass. Potential complications include headache, nerve root or conus medullaris damage, brain herniation, meningitis and bleeding. A standard approach is listed below:

Condition and natural history
Options and alternatives
Name of procedure; Not to treat
Side-effects
Extra procedures
Named person operating
Trial and Training (i.e. research and students)
Second opinion

Consolidation

Reiterate the key points of this consultation. Allow time to address any concerns or questions that Mrs Lee may have. Finally, ask her to sign the consent form.

Conclusion

Provide Mrs Lee with a copy of her consent form and an information leaflet. You should also provide her with your own contact information.

Case 7: Complaint

As the surgical trainee, you are required to review Miss Bradstone following her varicose vein surgery. She has been waiting for 4 hours for your decision as to whether she may be discharged home. Miss Bradstone is upset and unaware that you have been unavoidably delayed in surgery.

Preparation

Ensure that you have read the patient's medical, operative and nursing notes and confirmed the diagnosis. Ensure that you speak to Miss Bradstone in a private and calm environment and have the patient's nurse present.

Introduction

A full introduction is required.

Consultation

Acknowledge that Miss Bradstone has been kept waiting, and apologise. Explain your unavoidable delay and assure her that you will do your best to rectify the situation. Show empathy. Explain that after you have examined her you will make a final decision regarding her discharge.

Consolidation

Reiterate the key points of this consultation. Allow time to address any concerns or questions that the patient may have.

Conclusion

Provide Miss Bradstone with a clear management plan. Establish when further information will be available. Provide your own contact details.

Case 8: Complaint

As the junior surgical trainee, you are required to review Mr Miller, who has been admitted with acute appendicitis and is listed for emergency surgery. However, his operation has been delayed for the last 7 hours due to the admission of a trauma patient. In addition, there will be another unavoidable delay because a patient with a ruptured aortic aneurysm has just been taken to theatre.

Preparation

Ensure that you have read the patient's medical notes and confirmed the diagnosis. Ensure that you speak to Mr Miller in a private and calm environment and have the patient's nurse present.

Introduction

A full introduction is required.

Consultation

Acknowledge that Mr Miller has been kept waiting, and apologise. Explain the unavoidable delay, and assure him that you will do your best to rectify the situation. Show empathy. Explain the reasons for the delay, and ensure that Mr Miller's operation will be performed as soon as possible.

Consolidation

Reiterate the key points of this consultation. Allow time to address any concerns or questions that the patient may have.

Conclusion

Provide Mr Miller with a clear management plan. Establish when further information will be available. Provide your own contact details.

Case 9: Complaint

As the surgical trainee, you are required to review Mr Patel, who underwent an elective lumbar laminectomy. During the operation, he sustained a CSF leak and is required to lie flat in bed for two days. The patient's surgical wound is red, hot, tender and discharging fluid. Mr Patel complains of pain and that this operation has 'gone wrong.' He demands to speak to the consultant, who is currently unavailable.

Preparation

In this case, it is essential to read the patient's medical, operative and nursing notes to confirm the complication and the post-operative instructions. Ensure that you speak to Mr Patel in a private and calm environment, and have the patient's nurse present.

Introduction

A full introduction is required. Apologise, and explain that the consultant is not available at the moment. Ensure that Mr Patel is aware that you can fully address his concerns.

Consultation

Listen carefully to all of Mr Patel's complaints. Show empathy. Explain that his condition is one of the unfortunate possible complications of a lumbar laminectomy. Reassure Mr Patel that his operation was successful and that the CSF leak and infection are being treated. Tell him that he will soon 'feel better.'

Consolidation

Reiterate the key points of this consultation. Allow time to address any concerns or questions that the patient may have.

Conclusion

Provide Mr Patel with a clear management plan and arrange for a further meeting with the consultant. Establish when further information will be available. Provide the patient with your own contact details.

Clinical scenarios: information gathering

Case 1: Superficial lesion – skin nodule

Mr Terry, an 81-year-old man, presents with a non-tender skin lesion on his face. He attends clinic with his wife.

Preparation

Ensure that you have read Mr Terry's referral letter.

Introduction

Introduce yourself to Mr Terry and his wife. Establish good eye contact.

Consultation

Obtain Mr Terry's history using a standard approach as follows:

Personal details
Name, age, occupation and ethnic origin of patient

Presenting complaint

History of presenting complaint (HPC)
- Presentation of symptoms (acute or gradual), duration, location, size, progression, relieving and aggravating factors, colour, position, tenderness, discharge, quantity
- Systematic symptoms (i.e. weight loss, change in appetite, fevers)
- Risk factors (i.e. sun exposure, fair skin, X-rays, immunosuppression)
- Previous investigations and treatment

Past medical, surgical and anaesthetic history

Medication and allergies

Family history
Congenital disorders: basal-cell naevus, xeroderma pigmentosum

> **Social history**
> Marital status
> Occupation
> Smoking habits (number of pack years) and alcohol intake (units/week)
> Living accommodation
> Travel history (sun exposure)
>
> **Review of systems**

Consolidation

Reiterate the key points of Mr Terry's history. Allow time to address any concerns or questions that Mr and Mrs Terry may have.

Mr Terry wants to know what this lesion is and whether treatment is necessary.

Explain to Mr Terry that the lesion may represent a common skin cancer, called a basal-cell carcinoma. It is commonly found on the face of middle-aged to elderly fair people, and is twice as common in males. The lesion has been described as a 'rodent ulcer', as it is usually round with rolled, pearly edges. The centre of the lesion is ulcerated. It rarely spreads. The treatment of small lesions includes surgical excision and avoidance of sun exposure. In advanced cases, radiotherapy may be necessary.

Conclusion

Thank Mr Terry and now present his history to the examiner.

Case 2: Superficial lesions – groin lump

Mr Williams, a 32-year-old man, attends a Pre-Assessment Clinic for his upcoming operation (right-sided inguinal hernia repair). He is diabetic and takes regular insulin.

Preparation

Ensure that you have read Mr Williams' referral letter.

Introduction

Introduce yourself to Mr Williams. Establish good eye contact.

Personal details
Name, age, occupation and ethnic origin of patient

Presenting complaint

History of presenting complaint (HPC)
- Presentation of symptoms (acute or gradual), duration, size, position, progression, relieving and aggravating factors, tenderness, reducibility
- System-specific (gastrointestinal) questions (i.e. pain, masses, nausea, vomiting, regurgitation, dysphasia, distension, flatus, change in bowel habit, sphincter involvement, etc.)
- Systematic symptoms (i.e. weight loss, change in appetite, fevers, jaundice)
- Risk factors (i.e. cough, heavy lifting, constipation)
- Previous investigations and treatment

Past medical, surgical and anaesthetic history
As the patient is a known diabetic, it is important to establish his diabetic control and management. Ask to review his blood glucose diary, and ask him about any specific eye, kidney, nerve, foot and vascular complications.

Medication and allergies
Include insulin (slow- or long-acting), oral hypoglycaemics, aspirin, statins
(Explain that he may need to be admitted the night prior to surgery for an insulin sliding scale. If he takes aspirin, this should be stopped 1 week prior to surgery)

Family history

Social history
Marital status
Occupation
Smoking habits (number of pack years) and alcohol intake (units/week).
Living accommodation

Review of systems

Consultation

Obtain Mr Williams' history using a standard approach as follows:

Consolidation

Reiterate the key points of Mr Williams' history. Ensure that he understands the diagnosis (hernia, i.e. a protrusion of tissue through a weakness in the lower abdominal wall) and the operation (in this case, the procedure will be performed under general anaesthetic, and a small incision will be made over the hernia and the weakness in the abdominal wall will be repaired). Allow time to address any concerns or questions that he may have.

Conclusion

Thank Mr Williams and now present his history to the examiner.

Case 3: Musculoskeletal – hip pain

Mrs Khan, a 64-year-old woman, complains of right hip pain and difficulty in walking.

Preparation

Ensure that you have read Mrs Khan's referral letter.

Introduction

Introduce yourself to Mrs Khan. Establish good eye contact.

Consultation

Obtain Mrs Khan's history using a standard approach as follows:

Personal details
Name, age, occupation and ethnic origin of the patient

Presenting complaint

History of presenting complaint (HPC)
- Pain (muscle, bone or joint), deformity, swelling, stiffness, limb weakness, decreased range of movement, and functional loss. Specific to pain: Site, Onset, Character, Radiation, Associations, Timing and duration, Exacerbating and relieving factors, Severity

- Systematic symptoms (i.e. weight loss, night pain, fevers)
- Risk factors (i.e. trauma)
- Previous investigations and treatment

Past medical, surgical and anaesthetic history

Medication and allergies

Family history

Social history
Marital status
Occupation
Smoking habits (number of pack
years) and alcohol intake (units/week).
Living accommodation (i.e. house
or flat, including access)
Independence with regard to activities of daily living (ADL).

Review of systems

Consolidation
Reiterate the key points of Mrs Khan's history. Allow time to address any concerns or questions that she may have.

Mrs Khan states that she has difficulty in caring for her husband, who is recovering from surgery.

Assess Mrs Khan's level of independence and what home support she may require (through her own doctor, occupational therapist, physiotherapist and social services).

Conclusion
Thank Mrs Khan and now present her history to the examiner.

Case 4: Neurology – median nerve palsy and carpal tunnel syndrome

Mrs Hill, a 42-year-old woman, presents to clinic with pain and numbness in her hand. Recently she has been dropping objects, and she states that the pain is worse at night.

Preparation
Ensure that you have read Mrs Hill's referral letter.

Introduction
Introduce yourself to Mrs Hill. Establish good eye contact.

Consultation
Obtain Mrs Hill's history using a standard approach as follows:

Personal details
Name, age, occupation and ethnic origin of patient

Presenting complaint

History of presenting complaint (HPC)
- Pain (this may be referred beyond the cutaneous distribution of the median nerve), paraesthesia (lateral palm and lateral two and a half fingers), weakness, deformity, swelling, stiffness, decreased range of movement, functional loss. Specific to pain: Site, Onset, Character, Radiation, Associations, Timing and duration, Exacerbating and relieving factors, Severity
- Systematic symptoms (i.e. night pain)
- Risk factors (i.e. trauma, pregnancy, obesity)
- Previous investigations and treatment

Past medical, surgical and anaesthetic history
Myxoedema, acromegaly, rheumatoid arthritis, diabetes mellitus

Medication and allergies
Oral contraceptive pill

Family history

Social history
Marital status
Occupation and hazards (vibrating tools)
Smoking habits (number of pack years) and alcohol intake (units/week).
Living accommodation

Review of systems

Consolidation
Reiterate the key points of Mrs Hill's history. Allow time to address any concerns or questions that she may have.

Conclusion
Thank Mrs Hill and now present her history to the examiner.

Case 5: Circulatory – ulcer
Mr Broadman, a 78-year-old man, attends a Vascular Outpatients Clinic with a leg ulcer.

Preparation
Ensure that you have read Mr Broadman's referral letter.

Introduction
Introduce yourself to Mr Broadman. Establish good eye contact.

Consultation
Obtain Mr Broadman's history using a standard approach as follows:

Personal details
Name, age, occupation and ethnic origin of patient

Presenting complaint

History of presenting complaint (HPC)
- Presentation of symptoms (acute or gradual), duration, nature, progression, relieving and aggravating factors, colour, position, tenderness, discharge, quantity

- System-specific (vascular) questions: (i.e. chest pain, dyspnoea, orthopnoea, palpitations, dizziness, pain, leg/ankle swelling, etc.)
- Systematic symptoms (i.e. weight loss, change in appetite, fevers)
- Risk factors (i.e. trauma, diabetes mellitus)
- Previous investigations and treatment

Past medical, surgical and anaesthetic history
- *Venous ulcers: varicose veins or deep vein thrombosis*
- *Arterial ulcers: atheroma, Buerger's disease, rheumatoid arthritis*
- *Neuropathic ulcers: alcohol, diabetes*
- *Neoplastic ulcers: squamous-cell carcinoma (Marjolin's ulcer), basal-cell carcinoma or malignant melanoma*

Medication and allergies

Family history

Social history
Marital status
Occupation and associated hazards
Smoking habits (number of pack years) and alcohol intake (units/week).
Living accommodation

Review of systems

Consolidation
Reiterate the key points of Mr Broadman's history. Ensure that he understands his condition and its possible aetiology (venous, arterial, neuropathic, neoplastic or mixed). Allow time to address any concerns or questions that he may have.

Conclusion
Thank Mr Broadman and now present his history to the examiner.

Case 6: Circulatory – deep vein thrombosis

Miss Smithson, a 34-year-old woman, attends a Vascular Outpatients Clinic with a left swollen and painful calf.

Preparation

Ensure that you have read Miss Smithson's referral letter.

Introduction

Introduce yourself to Miss Smithson. Establish good eye contact.

Consultation

Obtain Miss Smithson's history using a standard approach as follows:

Personal details
Name, age, occupation and ethnic origin of patient

Presenting complaint

History of presenting complaint (HPC)
- Presentation of symptoms (acute or gradual), duration, progression, relieving and aggravating factors, unilateral/bilateral, pain, skin changes, colour, position. Specific to pain: Site, Onset, Character, Radiation, Associations, Timing and duration, Exacerbating and relieving factors, Severity
- System-specific (vascular) questions: (i.e. chest pain, dyspnoea, orthopnoea, palpitations, dizziness, pain, leg/ankle swelling, etc.)
- Systematic symptoms (i.e. weight loss, change in appetite, fevers)

Risk factors for DVT (Virchow's triad): blood flow (i.e. stasis), vessel wall (i.e. compression, trauma) and blood constituents (i.e. hyperviscosity, hypercoagulability)

Patient factors
Age > 40 years	*Female gender*
Pregnancy	*Obesity*
Oral contraceptive pill	*Previous DVT/PE*

Thrombophilia (protein C, protein S or factor V deficiencies)

Operative/pathological factors
Surgery duration > 150 minutes   *Laparoscopic procedure*
Post-operative immobility > 4 days   *Sepsis*
Major abdominal or pelvic surgery   *Malignancy*
Pelvic or long bone fracture

Previous investigations and treatment

Past medical, surgical and anaesthetic history

Medication and allergies

Family history

Social history
Marital status
Occupation and associated hazards
Smoking habits (number of pack years) and alcohol intake (units/week).
Living accommodation
Travel history (long-distance air travel)

Review of systems

Consolidation
Reiterate the key points of Miss Smithson's history. Ensure that she understands her condition. Allow time to address any concerns or questions that she may have.

Conclusion
Thank Miss Smithson and now present her history to the examiner.

Case 7: Trunk, abdomen – haematuria

Mr Howard, a 53-year-old man, attends the Urology Outpatients Clinic with painless haematuria.

Preparation

Ensure that you have read Mr Howard's referral letter.

Introduction

Introduce yourself to Mr Howard. Establish good eye contact.

Consultation

Obtain Mr Howard's history using a standard approach as follows:

Personal details
Name, age, occupation and ethnic origin of patient

Presenting complaint

History of presenting complaint (HPC)
- Presentation of symptoms (acute or gradual), duration, nature (macro- or microscopic), progression, relieving and aggravating factors, colour, consistency, quantity
- System-specific (gastrointestinal/urogenital) questions: (i.e. pain, masses, frequency, nocturia, dysuria, polyuria, urgency, sphincter involvement, etc.)
- Systematic symptoms (i.e. weight loss, change in appetite, fevers)
- Risk factors (i.e. trauma)
- Previous investigations and treatment

Past medical, surgical and anaesthetic history
Haematological conditions: sickle-cell anaemia

Medication and allergies
Anticoagulation: aspirin, clopidogrel, warfarin

Family history
Congenital conditions (polycystic kidney) and urological cancers (renal, bladder)

Social history
Marital status
Occupation and associated hazards
Smoking habits (number of pack years) and alcohol intake (units/ week).
Living accommodation
Travel history (schistosomiasis)

Review of systems

Consolidation
Reiterate the key points of Mr Howard's history. Allow time to address any concerns or questions that he may have.

Conclusion
Thank Mr Howard and now present his history to the examiner.

Case 8: Trunk, abdomen – rectal bleeding
Mrs Lewis, a 49-year-old woman, presents with a history of rectal bleeding for the last 2 months. She has been referred by her general practitioner for further investigation.

Preparation
Ensure that you have read Mrs Lewis's referral letter.

Introduction
Introduce yourself to Mrs Lewis. Establish good eye contact.

Consultation
Obtain Mrs Lewis's history using a standard approach as follows:

Personal details
Name, age, occupation and ethnic origin of patient

Presenting complaint

History of presenting complaint (HPC)
- Presentation of symptoms (acute or gradual), duration, nature, progression, relieving and aggravating factors, colour, consistency, quantity
- System-specific (gastrointestinal) questions: (i.e. pain, masses, nausea, vomiting, regurgitation, dysphasia, distension, flatus, change in bowel habit, sphincter involvement, etc.)
- Systematic symptoms (i.e. weight loss, change in appetite, fevers, jaundice)
- Risk factors (i.e. trauma, anticoagulation)
- Previous investigations and treatment

Past medical, surgical and anaesthetic history

Medication and allergies

Family history
Previous bowel cancer, inflammatory bowel disease (including Crohn's disease and ulcerative colitis), congenital conditions (familial adenomatous polyposis)

Social history
Marital status
Occupation
Smoking habits (number of pack years) and alcohol intake (units/week).
Travel history
Living accommodation

Review of systems

Consolidation

Reiterate the key points of Mrs Lewis's history. Allow time to address any concerns or questions that she may have.

Conclusion

Thank Mrs Lewis and now present her history to the examiner.

Case 9: Trunk, respiratory – post-operative shortness of breath

Mrs Lacey, a 74-year-old woman, is day 3 post total knee replacement and presents with acute shortness of breath.

Preparation

Ensure that you have read Mrs Lacey's medical, operative and nursing notes.

Introduction

Introduce yourself to Mrs Lacey. Establish good eye contact.

Consultation

First, assess (and if necessary treat) Mrs Lacey according to the *Advanced Life Support Guidelines*:

Airway
Breathing
Circulation
Disability
Exposure

Then obtain Mrs Lacey's history using a standard approach as follows:

Personal details
Name, age, occupation and ethnic origin of patient

Presenting complaint

History of presenting complaint (HPC)
- Presentation of symptoms (acute or gradual), duration, nature, progression, relieving and aggravating factors
- System-specific (respiratory) questions: (i.e. pain, cough, sputum, haemoptysis, wheeze and hoarseness)

- Systematic symptoms (i.e. weight loss, change in appetite and fevers)
- Risk factors (immobility)
- Previous investigations and treatment

Past medical, surgical and anaesthetic history
COPD, asthma, myocardial infarction

Medication and allergies
Anticoagulation, TED stockings, bronchodilators, steroids, oxygen

Family history

Social history
Marital status
Occupation
Smoking habits (number of pack years) and alcohol intake (units/week)
Travel history (i.e. TB exposure)
Living accommodation

Consolidation

Reiterate the key points of Mrs Lacey's history. Ensure that she understands that acute shortness of breath in post-operative patients may represent a pulmonary embolism secondary to a deep venous thrombosis, pulmonary oedema or pneumonia, and warrants further investigation. Allow time to address any concerns or questions that she may have.

Conclusion

Thank Mrs Lacey and now present her history to the examiner.

Appendix 1: MRCS clinical course – mock exam score sheet

	Superficial lesions	Abdomen/trunk	Musculoskeletal/neurological	Circulation
Attitudes				
Introduction	1 2 3 4	1 2 3 4	1 2 3 4	1 2 3 4
Patient interaction	1 2 3 4	1 2 3 4	1 2 3 4	1 2 3 4
Professional interaction	1 2 3 4	1 2 3 4	1 2 3 4	1 2 3 4
Clinical skills				
Gentleness of handling	1 2 3 4	1 2 3 4	1 2 3 4	1 2 3 4
Organisation of approach	1 2 3 4	1 2 3 4	1 2 3 4	1 2 3 4
General assessment	1 2 3 4	1 2 3 4	1 2 3 4	1 2 3 4
Inspection	1 2 3 4	1 2 3 4	1 2 3 4	1 2 3 4
Palpation	1 2 3 4	1 2 3 4	1 2 3 4	1 2 3 4
Other relevant assessments	1 2 3 4	1 2 3 4	1 2 3 4	1 2 3 4
Identification of clinical signs	1 2 3 4	1 2 3 4	1 2 3 4	1 2 3 4
Knowledge				
Differential diagnosis	1 2 3 4	1 2 3 4	1 2 3 4	1 2 3 4
Management plan	1 2 3 4	1 2 3 4	1 2 3 4	1 2 3 4
Final score	1 2 3 4	1 2 3 4	1 2 3 4	1 2 3 4

Appendix 2: Insider's top 10 key cases

Superficial lesions
1 Ganglion
2 Lipoma
3 Sebaceous cyst
4 SCCs and BCCs
5 Keratoacanthoma
6 Seborrhoeic keratosis
7 Malignant melanoma
8 Thyroid lumps
9 Salivary gland swellings
10 Cervical lymphadenopathy

Orthopaedics and neurology
1 Osteoarthritis of hip/knee
2 Osteoarthritis of hands
3 Rheumatoid hands
4 Carpal tunnel syndrome
5 Dupuytren's contracture
6 Radial/median/ulnar nerve palsy
7 Mallet finger/toes
8 Hallux valgus
9 Disc prolapse
10 Winging scapula

Vascular

1 Ulcers – venous/ischaemic/neuropathic
2 Varicose veins
3 Diabetic foot
4 Ischaemic limb
5 Amputations
6 CABG
7 Aneurysms – AAA/femoral/popliteal
8 Raynaud's syndrome
9 Arteriovenous fistula
10 Gangrene

Abdomen and trunk

1 Groin hernia
2 Incisional and umbilical hernia
3 Hepatomegaly
4 Splenomegaly
5 Stoma
6 Scrotal lumps (hydrocoele/varicocele/epididymal cyst)
7 Transplanted kidney
8 Breast lump
9 Jaundice
10 Ascites

Appendix 3: Nerve lesions

Remember that nerves can also be injured by diabetes mellitus, ischaemia, vitamin B_{12} deficiency, etc.

Radial nerve

In axilla (very high lesion):

- Saturday-night palsy – neuropraxia from sleeping with arm over back of chair.
- Ill-fitting crutches (crutch palsy).
- Penetrating wounds in axilla or arm.

Mid humerus (high lesion):

- Fracture of humerus in its middle third (triceps spared, BR often spared).
- Tourniquet palsies.

(Triceps is weak if the radial nerve is injured above the junction of the upper and middle thirds of the humerus.)

(BR is weak if the radial nerve is injured in the middle third of the humerus or above.)

At or below elbow (low lesions):

- Elbow dislocations.
- Monteggia fracture dislocation.
- Ganglions.
- Surgical trauma/local wound.

Posterior interosseous nerve syndrome (entrapment of the nerve as it passes between the two heads of supinator under the *arcade of Frohse*, a thickening at the proximal edge of supinator) – no sensory loss, no wrist drop (ECRL not paralysed), hand held in radial deviation when attempting extension, unable to extend fingers against resistance at MCPJs (paralysis of extensor digitorum). Sometimes seen after operation at the proximal end of the radius, and may also be caused by swellings (lipoma, ganglion, synovial proliferation) in or around the radial tunnel. Resisted active supination of forearm with elbow in extension tightens the arcade of Frohse, reproducing symptoms.

Superficial radial nerve injury (*Wartenberg's syndrome*) – no motor loss, only sensory loss. Caused by entrapment of nerve beneath the brachioradialis. Sometimes severed in operations on the synovial extensor tendons of the thumb, as in an operation for De Quervain's syndrome. Pain from nerve injury can be localised, and must be distinguished from conditions such as De Quervain's syndrome.

Radial tunnel syndrome – like posterior interosseous nerve syndrome, radial tunnel syndrome is considered to be the result of entrapment of the posterior interosseous nerve. Radial tunnel syndrome may represent an early posterior interosseous nerve syndrome. However, the distinction is useful because in radial tunnel syndrome, in contrast to posterior interosseous nerve syndrome, no motor deficits are observed. Patients typically present with pain over the lateral forearm with repetitive elbow extension and forearm rotation. This is frequently misdiagnosed as lateral epicondylitis.

Ulnar nerve

Ulnar tunnel syndrome (Guyon's canal or piso-hamate tunnel):

- Ganglion, lipoma.
- Fracture of the hook of hamate.
- Irritation from arthritic piso-triquetral joint.
- Repeated trauma over the hypothenar area.
- Ulnar artery aneurysm.

At wrist:

- Occupational trauma.
- Lacerations.
- Ganglia.

Distal to elbow:

- Compression as it passes through two heads of the FCU.

Level of medial epicondyle (cubital tunnel syndrome), most commonly, where nerve is very superficial:

▶ Usually idiopathic.
▶ Trauma (fracture of medial epicondyle, or compression from resulting callus).
▶ Local friction (prolonged pressure in anaesthetised patients on the operating table).
▶ Pressure.
▶ Stretching in long-standing cubitus valgus (tardy ulnar syndrome) or osteophytic spur in OA.
▶ *Fascial arcade of Struthers.*
▶ Exostoses from medial epicondyle.
▶ Hypertrophied synovium.
▶ Medial intermuscular septum itself.
▶ Osbourne's fascia – a fascial band bridging the two heads of the FCU.
▶ Accessory muscle – anconeus epitrochlearis.
▶ Ganglion.

High lesions:

▶ After supracondylar fracture, elbow dislocations, fractures.
▶ As part of a brachial plexus injury due to trauma.
▶ Compression secondary to a cervical rib.

Median nerve

Carpal tunnel, most commonly:

▶ Carpal tunnel syndrome, usually idiopathic.

Wrist:

▶ Lacerations.
▶ Dislocation of carpal lunate.
▶ Colles' fracture.

Forearm:

▶ Anterior interosseous nerve injury from forearm bone fractures, isolated neuritis or compression band.

Distal to elbow:

▶ Pronator teres entrapment syndrome (*ligament of Struthers*, which is a connection between the medial epicondyle and humerus or arch-like origin of the pronator teres or FDS).

Elbow:
- Dislocation.
- Supracondylar fracture.

Pronator syndrome – presents similarly to carpal tunnel syndrome, but the skin over the thenar eminence will be numb, and there is dull pain present in the proximal forearm (accentuated by use). Pain is reproduced by testing pronation against resistance.

Anterior interosseous nerve syndrome – the anterior interosseous nerve can be selectively compressed. There is motor weakness without sensory symptoms. The patient is unable to make the 'OK' sign (i.e. pinching with the thumb and index finger joint flexed, like a ring) because of weakness of the flexor pollicis longus and flexor digitorum profundus to the index finger (*see* Figure 1, p.57).

Appendix 4: Myotomes and dermatomes

Upper limb myotomes
- Shoulder abduction: C5 (deltoids and supraspinatus, axillary and suprascapular n).
- Shoulder adduction: C6/7 (pectoral and latissimus dorsi, medial and lateral pectoral n, thoracodorsal n).
- Elbow flexion: C5/6 (biceps and brachialis, musculocutaneous n).
- Elbow extension: C7/8 (triceps, radial n).
- Wrist extension: C6/7 (long forearm extensors, radial n).
- Wrist flexion: C6/7 (long forearm flexors, median and ulnar n).
- Finger flexion: C7/8 (long and short finger flexors, median and ulnar n).
- Finger extension: C7/8 (long and short finger extensors, radial n).
- Finger abduction: C8/T1 (dorsal interossei, ulnar n).
- Finger adduction: C8/T1 (palmar interossei, ulnar n).
- Thumb abduction: C8/T1 (abductor pollicis brevis, median n).
- Thumb adduction: C8/T1 (adductor pollicis, ulnar n).
- 'OK' sign: C8/T1 (FPL and FDP, anterior interosseous n) (*see* Figure 1, p.57).

Lower limb myotomes
- Hip flexion: L2/3 (iliopsoas, lumbar plexus and femoral n).
- Hip extension: L5/S1 (gluteus maximus, inferior gluteal n).
- Knee extension: L3/4 (quadriceps, femoral n).
- Knee flexion: L5/S1 (hamstrings, sciatic n).

- Ankle dorsiflexion: L4/5 (tibialis anterior and long extensors, deep peroneal n).
- Ankle plantar flexion: S1/2 (gastrocnemius and soleus, sciatic n).
- Foot inversion: L5/S1 (tibialis anterior and posterior, deep peroneal and tibial n).
- Foot eversion: L5/S1 (peronei, superficial peroneal n).
- Hallux extension: L5 (extensor hallucis longus, deep peroneal n).
- Toe flexion: S1/2 (flexor digitorum/hallucis longus, tibial n).

Upper limb dermatomes

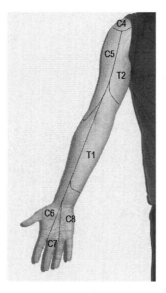

Figure A4a: Upper limb dermatomes (anterior).

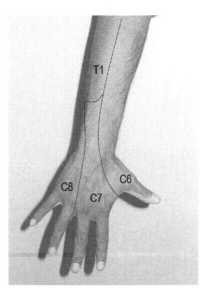

Figure A4b: Upper limb dermatomes (posterior).

Lower limb dermatomes

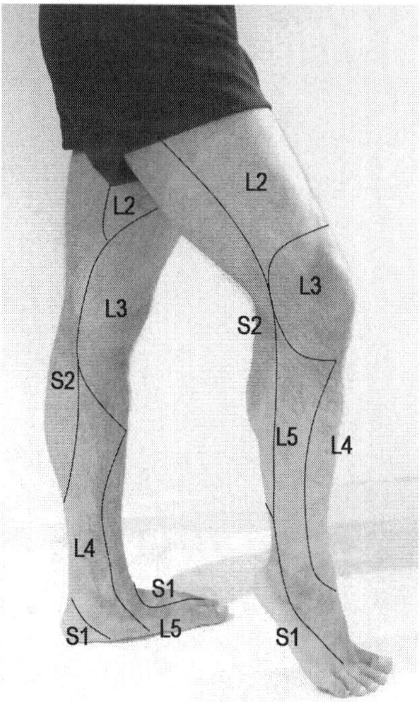

Figure A4c: Lower limb dermatomes.

Index